ONE NURSE AT A TIME:

Lessons Learned

*True Stories of Humanitarian
Responders on the Front Line*

Edited by Amanda Judd

Hendrix College Odyssey Program Editorial Assistants:
Jacie Andrews, Michelle DeLouise-Ashmore, Lily Bay, Bailey
Brya, Peyton Coffman, Leah Crenshaw, Zelda Engeler-Young,
Oliver Kuhns, Peyton Penny, Sarah Weems, Jasmine Zandi

Hand Heart Cover Art: Jacie Andrews and Peyton Coffman

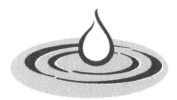

One Nurse At A Time is a non-profit organization that helps nurses become involved in volunteer work. We believe that nurses are pebbles, which, when dropped into the pond, make far-reaching ripples. If we can put more nurses into the world, we will exponentially impact healthcare for those most in need.

For more information, please go to
www.OneNurseAtATime.org

To contact us for speaking events, book clubs, or questions about volunteering: OneNurseAtATime@gmail.com

Also Available:

One Nurse At A Time: Beyond Borders: Humanitarian Nursing at the Edge of the World. Edited by Sue Averill RN

One Nurse At A Time: On a Mission: A Personal Journey into the Heart of Humanitarian Nursing By Sue Averill and Elizabeth Coulter

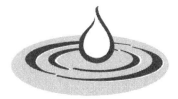

ISBN: 978-0-9977325-2-8

Dedicated to humanitarian workers who spend their own lives in the service of others.

Contents

Introduction

At One Nurse At A Time, we have reflected on our diverse and varied experiences in humanitarian work. Some of us began doing this work in our youth, others later in life. Perhaps we had a desire to see the world. Others felt it was a calling. Regardless, we all wanted to help the underserved.

We began to realize that there are many romanticized stories of mission work, but very few stories that illustrate the challenges we face as humanitarian workers. In *Lessons Learned*, we attempt to explore what happens when things go wrong and what you can do to prevent mistakes from happening.

We know that using your skills, time, and money for the benefit of others is a fine and noble cause, but when is that not enough? Many of the stories you will read explore missions where things went wrong, how you can avoid our mistakes, how you cope, and what we learned.

In this book, you will find that some of the mission stories are so inspiring that you would never want to come home. Why would you? The impact that a humanitarian worker has can seem so much more immediate in desperate situations than at home. These stories are important. They are the reasons why we do what we do.

However, it is equally important to give your attention to the harder lessons. Lessons that force you to grow in your understanding of cultures, governments, development, the impact of wars and colonialism, safety, organizations, and bureaucracies. Lessons that help you see life through a different lens. Lessons that create more questions than answers.

As you grow in your humanitarian work, your perspectives will change, sometimes dramatically. You will learn that this work is not just about naively setting out on a mission wanting to save the world. It's about understanding the challenges of a population, educating yourself about global health, and understanding the ethics of humanitarian work. It's about knowing how to prepare before you go and what you are willing to risk.

So sit back, relax, maybe get a little uncomfortable, and reflect — perhaps even review the Reader's Guide. In this book, you will read stories told by nurses, non-medical workers, and, in one case, national staff. You will be transported to Uganda, Malawi, Guatemala, Zambia, and other locations around the world. Your journey will be heartwarming at times, and at others will test your beliefs about how the world should be.

Perhaps the most important lesson is that humanitarian work is all of these things. We simply have to figure out how to navigate the seas of challenges that come our way, all the while maintaining an understanding of why it is important that you do this work—the good work.

Amanda Judd
Denver, 2018

African Skies
Liza Leukhardt

I was seventeen years old when I started daydreaming about being a humanitarian worker in Africa. I was almost sixty when I finally set foot on the African continent for the first time. In my seventeen-year-old fantasies I was being driven across the savannah at a jaunty clip by my trusty assistant, zebra herds parting at my approach to some spectacularly colorful village where everyone knew and loved me because I had cured them all of some unnamed and horrible but not too messy disease. Heavy drums playing in the background, hordes of smiling children would greet me, although nobody too sweaty or sticky. My seventeen-year-old fantasies were fueled by whatever was available to me at the time: documentaries, records of African folk music, the television show *Daktari*, which I watched religiously. When I look back, I seem to have been a pretty hilarious dreamer, but somehow the seed was planted. That fantasy took many forms throughout my life, but steadfastly remained somewhere in my psyche.

Fast forward through my years of raising three children,

3

multiple careers, detours through illness, divorce, soul-searching, and spiritual awakening. I had entered nursing at forty with a joy that sprang from finally realizing a dream to work in the medical field with humanitarian intentions. Somewhere deep inside, that seventeen-year-old nerd was alive and well. An empty nest gave me the time to pursue yoga and meditation, perhaps a key to some insight. Approaching sixty is a good time for self-assessment and bucket lists. After twenty years working in hospice the universe gave me a good kick in the butt. "Go do what you always wanted to do. You can now; you're a nurse!"

2012 was the year I finally stepped onto African soil. How do I describe the pure joy I felt in finally realizing a life-long dream? Sitting in the back of a truck with my team mates, being driven from the airport to our living quarters in Monrovia, I couldn't stop grinning. There was a smell in the air, the wood smoke from cooking fires, which I've come to associate with developing countries. In the years since this trip, every time I smell wood smoke, my heart fills and I think of Africa.

Of course, I snapped out of all that romantic dreamy stuff pretty quickly. After a rest day it was time to travel. With my three teammates, our Liberian nursing assistant, our driver, two young female assistants, all our gear, suitcases full of donated medications and supplies, and our food for the week as well as a few live chickens, we squeaked into our Toyota truck like sardines in a tin. We were headed a little over a hundred miles away to a small remote village on the border with Guinea.

Pretty quickly, it was time to get to work. After many years of civil war there is very little infrastructure left in Liberia. Once we were off the main road through Monrovia, we hit nothing but dirt roads with potholes the size of moon craters. I have some pretty funny sideways videos where we tried to capture what it was like. After about five hours of smashing our heads against the windows, it wasn't funny anymore. Of course, with those kinds of roads our ancient truck had multiple breakdowns. After the third one, we landed in a village for several hours while all the men stared at the wheels with hopeless expressions and shrugged while the women made peanut butter sandwiches. I managed to get a dressing on the open leg wound of a wiggly, screaming toddler, which made me feel very professional. Little did I know that in the following week I would probably do hundreds of those dressings.

After being thrown around the back of the truck for fourteen hours, we made it to the village. By then, we may have all had concussions. Rain like I've never imagined was pouring down while we unpacked. We slept on foam mats on concrete floors. The outhouse was a very long, wet walk across the street and we were instructed never to go alone. Like a row of ducklings, we all slogged down there together. One of my teammates emerged with toilet paper stuffed into her nostrils.

The next day, we packed the truck up with all our supplies at the crack of dawn. Hurrah! Finally, we arrived at a clinic! Even though we were in a remote village already, we were going to a yet more remote village in Guinea. People, we were told, had walked all night to get there and were already waiting. The rainy season had just ended, and our driver eyed the knee-deep mud on the road doubtfully. We probably drove about five-hundred feet before we got thoroughly, up-to-the-tires stuck. A little voice in my head said, "We can have clinic here. Isn't this remote enough?" After a quick conference it was decided that we would walk to the village, carrying all our stuff, since it was "only" seven kilometers away.

By the time I had shouldered my backpack, a new development came along. A group of young men from the village careened down the hill on dirt bikes, buzzing like dragonflies through the mud, offering to help. Overcome by simultaneous feelings of absolute terror and "how cool is this?", I hoisted myself onto the back of a dirt bike, turned my baseball cap backwards, and clung for dear life to the kid driving. The urge to let out a manic Tarzan whoop possessed me as we went flying through the mud. This was infinitely better than my daydreams!

It still took a while for the whole team and all our stuff to get to the village via dirt bike. By then there were hundreds of very restless people waiting, and only four of us to provide whatever medical care we could. Somehow I became the designated wound care nurse, and the day passed in a blur as I treated the chronic sores and infections that come from living in an environment of dirt floors and poor hygiene.

My body sore from squatting and kneeling all day to look at legs and feet, I hauled myself on the back of the dirt bike. I squished between the driver in front and my teammate behind me, neither of us the most petite of women. Down the hill we went, the driver negotiating the muddy ruts with difficulty. As we leaned into a turn the kid lost control entirely, throwing the three of us into the mud.

I managed a quick inventory of my pathetic sixty-year-old body. Fingers and toes could wiggle, arms and legs were mobile. I was covered in mud, bruised, and sore as hell, thanking my lucky stars that I hadn't fractured a hip in the middle of nowhere. Somewhere in that mud was my flashlight, a valuable resource in a place with no electricity. Even in my hiking boots, mud squished between my toes, caked as far as my ankles, and speckled my glasses. A bucket bath in an unfinished cement room reeking of pee was the best I could look forward to for cleaning up, and, oh, did I look forward to it!

Once I returned to the room I shared mattress to mattress with my two female teammates, I made the mistake of sitting down, which led to lying down, which led to blissfully passing out.

"Hey Liza! Where are you? Are you sleeping?" I pretended not to hear. Maybe if I appeared totally unconscious she'd leave me alone. I felt a foot poking me in the ribs.

"Are you alive? I promised we would do an evening clinic in this village before the sun goes down." As I sat up, whatever was left of the romantic African daydream of my youth slowly evaporated. Setting up another clinic meant unpacking all our supplies and meds, setting up another pharmacy wherever we could find anything resembling a table, making a place for assessments, and working with a headlamp as the daylight faded. When the villagers heard a clinic was happening, the building instantly filled with chattering women, their babies tied to their backs, screaming children, and stoic elderly. Everyone had wounds and skin issues, yet I eked enough dressings and ointments out of my dwindling supplies to deal with them all.

Later, much later it seemed, I skipped dinner to go face-plant on my foam mattress, only to wake in the middle of the night to my two giggling teammates. "Is she breathing?" A goat bleated endlessly right outside the window then suddenly shrieked hideously and became silent. "I think a dinosaur ate the goat," my roommate commented. This, of course, sent us into fits of hysterical giggling, which led us to needing to pee. Because we females were not allowed out alone, we woke up our male colleague who was sleeping in another room and all traipsed across the street to the outhouse. We decided to have an impromptu team meeting while we took turns in the outhouse.

With no electricity for miles, the African sky was spectacular filled with brilliant stars and the light of the Milky Way. The village was absolutely silent. Ducks and chickens roosted in the corners. As I stood there exhausted, aching, and filthy, my heart filled with a profound gratitude and joy, yes, joy to be here in this place, in this perfect moment, with these perfect human beings. It was a feeling all too rare in life, when body, mind and spirit finally line up with the universe, with long cherished dreams and your reason for being here, on this planet, at this time.

The Road of Good Intentions

Christine VanHorn

Brightly beaded macramé jewelry adorned a square of blue fabric on the sidewalk near our hotel. An older Mayan woman had arrived before dawn and patiently waited on a three-legged wooden stool. As our team tumbled from our rooms, her smile greeted us, and she gestured to her goods. My fellow team members offered a cheery "Good Morning!" as they walked past her and boarded the bus. Our day began with a prayer, eggs and bread, and local coffee at a nearby church.

For years I had envied nurses who returned to the hospital where I work, bubbling over with stories from their medical missions. Their social media posts, pictures of them posing with young children from around the world, shouted, "Make the world a better place simply by showing up!" Having no medical background, I envisioned myself rocking babies in an orphanage and dreamed of enriching their lives with my presence. I wanted to save the poor children of the world, too!

Thinking to minimize culture shock, I googled "missions to English speaking countries," and Belize topped the list. The perfect place for a first mission! I found a non-profit organization to work with and convinced a few friends to join. My main concern was that I would not have a role on a medical mission, but I could practically *see* the babies waiting for me to hold and pat and coo to them.

Our old school bus, with seats built for children, bumped along dirt roads to our work site for the day. I peeled my sweaty shirt from the torn vinyl backrest and stiffly climbed out, rubbing my knees, bruised from banging against the seat-back in front of me.

Often, the only solid structure in a town was the church. We carried boxes and bags of supplies into the simple concrete building. We grouped pews into triage, consultation stations, and a waiting area. The altar was reverently moved aside and the pulpit turned into a pharmacy.

Those of us without medical backgrounds helped to set up and tear down, provided crowd control, and directed patients through the circuit. Midwest public health students taught hand hygiene and provided dental education. A local volunteer registered each patient into a laptop; the Belize Ministry of Health requires an electronic medical record for each patient. Although English is the official national language, most people in the rural areas speak one of the many Mayan dialects, and translators were essential.

Rather than rocking babies, I worked in the pharmacy, hand-writing each label with the name of the drug, how much to take, and how often. Vitamins and over-the-counter pain medications were staples, although some antibiotics and cough syrups were required.

I sought out the local helpers to ask about our patients. Although we were there during the rainy season, many people had traveled long distances by foot over muddy roads to come to our clinics. In the humid, 100-degree heat, the mosquitos were unbearable.

After each patient was seen and treated — up to a hundred in a six-hour day — we climbed tiredly onto the old school bus and made our way "home." Our modest hotel had running hot and cold water, electricity, WiFi, and air conditioning. Our patients waved us goodbye and walked away along the rain-soaked road. After a long shower and a quick email to my family, I kept thinking about the people we'd served that day and couldn't help but feel a pang of guilt.

Seeing so much poverty was eye-opening for me. This was not the American poverty of low-income housing, welfare, public health systems, and food stamps. These people were living in the jungle, far off the beaten path, in thatched-roof huts with dirt floors. This was subsistence living at best. They did not have cars. They walked everywhere and with luck were sometimes able to catch a bus to bigger towns and cities for work and trade. Young mothers carried their babies in modified slings strapped around their foreheads. At home, I take refrigeration for granted; here the indigenous population lived without it. I also found no flush toilets except at our hotel. Outhouses sported only a hole in the ground, and I learned to balance in a squat on my tiptoes. After the first time, I never forgot to keep tissues in my pocket. I was not prepared to experience lifestyles so vastly different from my own.

The older Mayan woman smiled to us from her stool each

morning as we purchased memories to take home. I asked a translator to help me hold a conversation with her. She was as curious about us as I was about her. On our last day, my new friend placed a string of beads around my neck and held my hands with a radiant smile. I wiped away my tears.

Since that first mission, I've read about and discussed the ethics of mission work extensively.

The organization we traveled with had a religious basis and was supported by local churches in Belize. Our mission was intended to be medical in nature and not evangelical. But even so, I was repeatedly asked by the people in the organization why I wasn't ministering to the American atheists in the group.

Medically speaking, there are a lot of groups that return to the same villages, following up with patients and teaming up with local doctors and nurses to build capacity. But this wasn't the case with our group. This organization had no plans to return or to follow up with these patients. There were no hospitals or clinics in the area, and another medical group might not come by for a year or more. So, I have to wonder, did we do any good at all?

As promised, there were a *lot* of children, constantly asking for toys and candy. I knew candy was not good in terms of diet and lack of dental care, but I wish that I had brought some small toys to share or even some bubbles to blow.

There were no orphan babies to cuddle and nurture. The explanation I was given is that Belize doesn't approve of foreigners visiting their orphanages. Once I was at home again, I began doing research and was shocked by what I discovered.

Orphanage tourism is an ethical minefield. Children with

living biological parents are often sent to these orphanages as a way to alleviate the burden of another mouth to feed and end up being a tourist attraction. Sometimes they are made to dance, entertain, and solicit funds from international volunteers. Volunteers rarely undergo background checks. They come for a short period of time, showering attention on the "orphans," leaving the children vulnerable to attachment disorders...or worse. I realized that my hope of rocking babies, although well-intended in my dreams, was potentially hazardous to those same children I wanted to nurture. Full-time staff was better for the little ones than my attentions would have been for one week.[1]

While I'm not sure our group had a lasting impact, I hold out hope that we did some good.

Reference list:

1. UNICEF. "With the Best Intentions: A Study of Attitudes Towards Residential Care in Cambodia." 2011, doi:https://www.unicef.org/eapro/Study_Attitudes_towards_R C.pdf.

The Problem with Little White Girls (and Boys): Why I Stopped Being a Voluntourist

Pippa Biddle

White people aren't told that the color of their skin is a problem very often. We sail through police checkpoints, don't garner sideways glances in affluent neighborhoods, and are generally understood to be predispositioned for success based on a physical characteristic (the color of our skin) we have little control over beyond sunscreen and tanning oil.

After six years of working in and traveling through a number of different countries where white people are in the numerical minority, I've come to realize that there is one place being white is not only a hindrance but negative – most of the developing world.

In high school, I traveled to Tanzania as part of a school trip. There were 14 white girls, 1 black girl who, to her frustration, was called white by almost everyone we met in Tanzania, and a few teachers/chaperones. $3000 bought us a week at an orphanage, a half-built library, and a few pickup soccer games, followed by a week-long safari.

Our mission while at the orphanage was to build a library. Turns out that we, a group of highly educated private boarding school students were so bad at the most basic construction work that each night the men had to take down the structurally unsound bricks we had laid and rebuild the structure so that, when we woke up in the morning, we would be unaware of our failure. It is likely that this was a daily ritual. Us mixing cement and laying bricks for 6+ hours, them undoing our work after the sunset, re-laying the bricks, and then acting as if nothing had happened so that the cycle could continue.

Basically, we failed at the sole purpose of our being there. It would have been more cost-effective, stimulative of the local economy, and efficient for the orphanage to take our money and hire locals to do the work, but there we were trying to build straight walls without a level.

That same summer, I started working in the Dominican Republic at a summer camp I helped organize for HIV+ children. Within days, it was obvious that my rudimentary Spanish set me so far apart from the local Dominican staff that I might as well have been an alien. Try caring for children who have a serious medical condition, and are not inclined to listen, in a language that you barely speak. It isn't easy. Now, 6 years later, I am much better at Spanish and am still highly involved with the camp programming, fundraising, and leadership. However, I have stopped attending having finally accepted that my presence is not the godsend I was coached by non-profits, documentaries, and service programs to believe it would be.

You see, the work we were doing in both the DR and Tanzania was good. The orphanage needed a library so that they could be accredited to a higher level as a school, and the camp in the DR needed funding and supplies so that it could provide HIV+ children with programs integral to their mental and physical health. It wasn't the work that was bad. It was me being there.

It turns out that I, a little white girl, am good at a lot of things. I am good at raising money, training volunteers, collecting items, coordinating programs, and telling stories. I am flexible, creative, and able to think on my feet. On paper I am, by most people's standards, highly qualified to do international aid. But I shouldn't be.

I am not a teacher, a doctor, a carpenter, a scientist, an engineer, or any other professional that could provide concrete support and long-term solutions to communities in developing countries. I am a 5′ 4″ white girl who can carry bags of moderately heavy stuff, horse around with kids, attempt to teach a class, tell the story of how I found myself (with accompanying powerpoint) to a few thousand people and not much else.

Some might say that that's enough. That as long as I go to X country with an open mind and a good heart I'll leave at least one child so uplifted and emboldened by my short stay that they will, for years, think of me every morning.

I don't want a little girl in Ghana, or Sri Lanka, or Indonesia to think of me when she wakes up each morning. I don't want her to thank me for her education or medical care or new clothes. Even if I am providing the funds to get the ball rolling, I want her to think about her teacher, community leader, or mother. I want her to have a hero who she can relate to – who looks like her, is part of her culture, speaks her language, and who she might bump into on the way to school one morning.

After my first trip to the Dominican Republic, I pledged to myself that we would, one day, have a camp run and executed by Dominicans. Now, about seven years later, the camp director, program leaders and all but a handful of counselors are Dominican. Each year we bring in a few Peace Corps Volunteers and highly-skilled volunteers from the USA who add value to our program, but they are not the ones in charge. I think we're finally doing aid right, and I'm not there.

Before you sign up for a volunteer trip anywhere in the world this summer, consider whether you possess the skill set necessary for that trip to be successful. If yes, awesome. If not, it might be a good idea to reconsider your trip. Sadly, taking part in international aid where you aren't particularly helpful is not benign. It's detrimental. It slows down positive growth and perpetuates the "white savior" complex that, for hundreds of years, has haunted both the countries we are trying to 'save' and our (more recently) own psyches. Be smart about traveling and strive to be informed and culturally aware. It's only through an understanding of the problems communities are facing, and the continued development of skills within that community, that long-term solutions will be created.

Used with permission of Pippa Biddle

The Burden

Dianne Thompson

Driving down the steep one-lane roads from the village, we sometimes saw blue morpho butterflies with giant, iridescent wings gliding along the sides of our vehicle. We saw them, that is, if it wasn't raining.

The United Methodist Volunteers in Mission had invited us to Guatemala. I had been twice before on other missions, but it was my husband's dream to go on a longer one, so here we were.

In most cases, mission teams are large groups of people with diverse skills, but back then, the team was more of a couple: my husband Jim and me. We were the *whole* team heading to Guatemala to renovate a building in the village of Paquila. The old structure had once been a clinic, but it was now abandoned except for bats, scorpions, and a few old boxes of maps and statistics.

Bordered by the Pacific Ocean to the south and dramatic volcanoes to the north, Paquila's heat and rough terrain lack the tourist appeal of the Mayan ruins of the Guatemalan lowlands or charm of the colonial towns of the Highlands. Frankly, it's the jungle. This tropical area of Guatemala is known as the Boca Costa. There's no wildlife except for the occasional iguana or snake, and empty armadillo shells decorate the modest homes.

During the rainy season, women walk across muddy roads, yards, and damp dirt floors in jelly shoes, and the elderly and young children go barefoot. Chickens and pigs forage through the village. It's not unusual to be kept up at night by the symphony of barking dogs, gently drifting off to sleep just as the rooster's crow reminds you that dawn is breaking.

Though the poverty is bleak, the locals' weaving and embroidery items are spectacular, detailed, and colorful. My eye was repeatedly drawn to the artwork in their woven blouses, called *huipiles* (we-peels). Most homes have a back strap loom hanging on a nail, waiting for the artisan to capture a story in her blouse's pattern.

We had planned to volunteer at this post for six months. As life goes, six months soon turned into six years, and after six years of juggling a mission in Guatemala with our lives back in the US, we built a house here and have called it home ever since. The Boca Costa Medical Mission (BCMM) was born out of this work.

There are so many stories, so many lives changed over the years, but there is one story that stands out.

I was out on a home visit when the eight-year-old girl arrived at the clinic. She had been carried quite a distance by her father. At the time, a doctor from the US was the volunteer physician on duty in the clinic. The little girl's abdomen was painfully distended with almost no bowel sounds – an ominous sign in the best of situations. The doctor did the best he could with what he knew and gave her some Milk of Magnesia and albendazole (dewormer). Clearly, he considered worms, but he didn't realize how severe it could be. He asked her to return the next day. The father agreed and left with the little girl in his arms.

Medical providers in developed countries have almost no training in recognizing a worm problem because developed countries have sanitation that makes these types of infections uncommon. It's easy to understand why the doctor may not have made the connection because in the US, when you see a cough, you never think worms. When you have decreased bowel sounds, you never think worms, but in the tropics, you must consider worms a possibility. At our BCMM clinic everyone had a stomach ache, a cough, diarrhea, head-to-toe itching, and anemia – all signs of parasitic infections and other diseases that present themselves in tropical climates. While the little girl had severe symptoms, the complaints were common in this part of the world.

Transmission of the ascariasis worm begins with the ingestion of eggs that then mature in the stomach, enter the circulation, and travel to the lungs. They are then coughed up and swallowed. In Paquila, all the right conditions exist for parasitic infections to develop: warmth, a humid climate, indiscriminate defecation of man and animal, moist soil, and poor sanitation and hygiene.

We're all familiar with gaggles of geese, swarms of bees, and parliaments of owls, but the presence of roundworms rampant in the intestinal tract or geographic area is known as a "burden." This burden of worms is a widespread condition, which in some rural areas can have an infection rate of greater than 90%.

I remained curious about what had happened to the little girl, so on one of my many home visits, I sought the family out.

When I arrived at her home, the father thanked us repeatedly for coming. He told us that he had seen a worm crawling out of her nose – a sure sign that the little girl's lack of bowel sounds was the result of a complete intestinal obstruction due to a burden. After leaving the clinic, he had carried the little girl over the mountainous terrain all the way home. She had died that night.

I lived with that story, the story of a completely preventable death.

I questioned why the doctor hadn't sent the little girl for an ultrasound and further testing. I questioned whether it would've made a difference if I had been at BCMM that day. I questioned and questioned, and in the end, I don't know if it would've changed the outcome for the little girl, but it changed a lot for us.

We began to look at what it would take to eradicate the burden.

The Guatemalan Ministry of Health had regulations in place to effectively eradicate the worm burden in their population. So why did Paquila and surrounding villages still have this problem? Was it the difficulty of accessing the rural areas? Was it the poverty? Was it because the people are indigenous Maya?

Whatever the reason, the areas we were serving were not being assisted.

We stopped asking why, and we started a regimented deworming program. We treated everyone equally. When asked if they had worms, a large majority said yes. So we administered the albendazole right there in our newly remodeled clinic in Paquila.

Our deworming program utilized a process similar to tuberculosis treatment in developing nations. Directly observed therapy (DOT) ensures that the patients are getting all of their medication and is a practical solution to partial treatments and "pill-saving" in developing countries with limited access to medication. Patients had to take all of the medicine in front of us and our small staff – DOT therapy.

This deworming program was so important that Jim and I sponsored the first village-wide deworming medicine program, along with the clinic's renovations, ourselves. Luckily, word got out, and teams of doctors and nurses soon began coming to work with us, bringing medications to replenish our supplies about every three months.

We dewormed thousands in Paquila and the surrounding villages. As we sustained this program, the burden was decreasing little by little. Manuel, Maria Elena, and Maria Coti, our local health care workers, documented the decrease in the burden in the twenty communities where we instituted the program.

It's hard to imagine how disproportionately parasitic infestations can affect the most disadvantaged, particularly in rural areas. These infections trap vulnerable communities in a cycle of poverty. Like the hookworm that used to be the scourge of Appalachia and the rural southern US, parasitic infestations cause malnutrition, stunted growth and development, and illness that decreases overall productivity.[1]

We now require enough albendazole and vitamins from each team to treat the 500+ patients who show up at the clinic when a team is present, and more importantly, enough for us to continue the effort between teams. We also ask that our medical teams, typically led by nurses, bring their own equipment. Deworming is an important task that should be integrated in missions throughout the tropics. It is very important to educate yourselves on diseases that are common where you are traveling. Your education could save a life!

These short-term mission teams are making a tremendous difference here in Guatemala. To those who are thinking of coming to serve — *you* are the life line. No one can convince us at Boca Costa that brief medical teams aren't worth the time.

Fifteen years later, the BCCM base clinic has become more sophisticated. Maria Elena became an auxiliary nurse and still works with us today. We have a dream team of permanent local nurses and health promoters.

Globally, success stories in village parasite control abound, but at the Boca Costa clinic the issue persists. The Guatemalan Ministry of Health says that the burden has been reduced by 80% in the villages we serve since the program's inception, but there are still untreated populations.

Everyone who comes to the clinic is still asked, "When did you last take an anti-parasite drug?" They shrug their shoulders, unsure. So we ask, "Do you want one?" They never refuse because they know. They *know* that there's an easy remedy to ease their burden.

Today, around the Boca Costa, kids are consistently attending school, and the outlook on education is different. Teachers are working with kids who no longer sit half asleep in their seats due to hunger and vitamin deficiencies. There are organized activities and sports where whole families attend, offering them a chance to socialize, learn from one another, and realize a more positive future for themselves.

And the nurses, those who dedicate their lives to global health work, those who spend their own money and use their vacations to care for people in a forgotten part of the world, what should we call them? A gaggle, a swarm? Surely, we know they are a *force*.

Reference list:

1. Nuwer, Rachel. "How a Worm Gave the South a Bad Name." *PBS*, Public Broadcasting Service, 27 Apr. 2016, www.pbs.org/wgbh/nova/next/nature/how-a-worm-gave-the-south-a-bad-name/.

The Story of a Birth: Zambia, Africa

Devorah Goldberg

The vast expanse of sky above the G'Nombe Clinic blanketed multitudes of people and herds of children, all pushing to clutch my hand, feel my curls, and even jump on me to get a selfie. There is nothing these children wouldn't do for a sweet, and it was seldom that I didn't give in.

I spent the daytime hours screening hundreds of children for their basic health assessment, the language barrier creating unexpected challenges in trying to address the maladies of last year, yesterday, or even "tomorrow." Understanding the terminology that the patients used went beyond my scope of practice as a nurse and even the knowledge gained in my nurse practitioner degree program to find a differential for "headaches on my knee", but a basic interpreter would have helped.

I've listened to hundreds of heartbeats and heard so many arrhythmias that I can orchestrate an intricate tune. I've looked into hundreds of ears and seen landscapes of wax, dirt, and often insects lining the ear canals, paving a bumpy, odorous road to the frequently infected eardrum. Examining their mouths as part of our general screening was a visual venture into the tunnels and pot holes of the cavities and rotten teeth scattered within their gums. Sometimes the case was a large hernia, other times an interesting rash or an infectious disease, but each day there was something we came home talking about. I looked into hundreds of eyes, each one deep, dark, and soulful with a life, with a story, with aches and pains that I didn't always understand.

I spent nighttime in Zambia awake, working in the labor ward. Why sleep when you are a night shift nurse at home?

The G'Nombe Clinic labor ward has a few clients: one is in active labor, one has been having contractions all day, but with no progress, and one mom needs IV fluids. I offer to place an IV, but the clinic is out of IV bags. We send the patient's mom and aunt to buy some drinks, and we give her oral rehydration. We encourage her to continue walking in hopes of progressing her scattered contractions into active labor. Another mom is in preterm labor at 26 weeks, so we have called an ambulance to come take her to hospital; 45 minutes later we are still waiting.

Soon another mom shows up. Her name is Giveness, and she is expecting her fourth child. She says that she has had pains since 1000. It is now 0300. Lacking proper electricity, the lighting in the clinic relies on a combination of solar powered lamps that work intermittently, candles, and the headlamp I brought from America. We perform a pelvic exam. There are no monitors to attach to Giveness, so we use a manual fetoscope that we place on her abdomen to measure the fetal heart rate. The midwife does an internal exam and determines that Giveness is fully dilated. It has been about 10 minutes since she arrived in the clinic; it's time to deliver the baby.

One of the lamps is beginning to dim. I pull out my headlamp, the midwife lights some candles, and we prepare the delivery equipment.

There is no such thing as pain medication or epidurals in this birthing ward. No machine adjusts Giveness's bed's height to convenience her body and its huge, painful abdomen. She climbs onto the bed on her own. We layer the bed with plastic garbage bag that Giveness brought from home and with her "Chitenga," a traditional linen that has a multitude of uses as skirts, dresses, hair wraps, and baby carriers. Here it is used to dress the bed that she will deliver her baby on. We layer the broken infant warmer with blankets brought from home to keep the newborn warm.

The midwives and I don our gloves and aprons, and we are ready to deliver. Giveness climbs onto the bed. There are no stirrups to secure her position. I hold on one side and the midwife assists with the other. She has no family there for moral support, so she squeezes my hand with every push. The baby is crowning.

The midwife turns to me, "Sister Devorah, are you ready to deliver a baby?" The last time that I had delivered a baby was a year prior in pure candlelight, in this very clinic, with the same midwife, Mwamba. However, what has changed in the past year is now we have some light, I have done this before, and I have become an ER nurse. I have learned that I must always be ready to deal with the unexpected.

Giveness begins to push, and she is definitely in pain, but she doesn't make a peep. The bed is flat, there are no pillows, and she is lying on her back, so we hold her legs. She holds up her own head as she pushes. Before I can blink, the head is out, and I begin to position it and guide the shoulders. The umbilical cord is wrapped loosely around the neck. I fumble my fingers through it and hold it down as the midwife helps pull the baby out. It is a tight squeeze. We dry her off with a towel and she yells out - strong, loud, shrill - and we place her on her mother for skin to skin. I give a proud sigh of relief. We are done; a new life is born. I clamp and cut the cord with a sharp needle because the razors they usually use are out of stock. With a candle still flickering in the background, I hold the baby up to Giveness so that she can see the miracle that she just bravely delivered.

It's a girl!

I mention to the midwife that the cord seems a bit short. She looks at the cord, touches the Giveness's still-firm belly, and says, "Sister, there is another." I quickly take what has now become Baby Number 1, weigh her (2.0kg), wrap her in blankets, and head back to the mom.

Giveness is not aware there have been not one, but two humans growing inside of her. When we used the fetoscope to listen to the heartbeat, we didn't think to listen for another. As Mwamba does an internal exam, she says that she feels a limb and the baby is in a breach position. However, because the fetal membranes are still intact, and we have no ultrasound or other diagnostic tools to assist us, she has difficulty determining the baby's exact position. She wants to place a urinary catheter because she needs an empty bladder to allow for more space to assess Giveness and maybe reposition the baby internally. Slight bump in the road: we are out of catheters. Mwamba thinks fast and grabs the IV tubing we had out for the mom who needed fluids. She tears the tube and places it inside the urethra as she would a catheter. The bladder drains, and she begins an internal exam.

Before we can do anything else, Giveness gives a strong push, and I look down to see what looks like a butt and a tiny hand. The little girl, Baby Number 2, makes her surprise entrance into the world, butt first!

We search for the other arm to pull out, and Giveness continues the hard work of pushing. Soon, the head is revealed with the cord around the neck. We untangle it and perform aggressive suction until Baby Number 2 reveals her voice — and ability to breathe — with a loud cry. Now, we breathe.

As I fumble to find oxygen and tend to the babies, Mwamba tends to the mom, delivering the placentas, stitching her up. Baby Number 2 weighs 2.1kg.

One of the overhead lamps that was flickering suddenly comes back to life with a brighter shine. Once Giveness is stitched up and cleaned, she gets up, carries her bucket of belongings, and sets herself up in the postpartum room. A short while later, after we have cleaned, dressed, and wrapped up her babies in layers of blankets and mini towels as diapers, the mom rests in bed, sheltered by her mosquito net. We hand her the babies to be fed and stay with her for the next few hours until she goes home.

There are no cribs in the postpartum room. The babies all sleep with the moms in the same bed, and Giveness and her babies are no different. They lie resting and tired in the postpartum room. Most mothers stay in the postpartum room for six hours until they are discharged, but since it is late at night,

Giveness will stay until the morning.

We now refocus our attention on the other laboring moms. The ambulance finally came to retrieve the woman in preterm labor, an hour and a half after it was called. We reassess the dehydrated mom who has been drinking fluids, and she is more dilated. Success! Labor is progressing. We allow her to continue resting and walking in the postpartum area until she is ready to push. We can't bring her to the delivery area, because both beds have been filled by other soon-to-be mothers who have just walked in in active labor.

It's nearly 0500. The midwives of G'Nombe Clinic didn't get to jump into their on-call bunk beds for a nap tonight because it was just too busy. As the sun begins to rise, two more babies are born. One of those babies is born in the postpartum area; our lady with the slow labor progression caught up rather quickly.

I head out of the compound just as the roosters are crowing their morning tunes. The sun is beating strongly. Patients begin to flood the lines of G'Nombe Clinic, and a new day has begun in a little compound in Zambia, Africa.

Approach and Landing
Elise Peterson

In the 1930s, the aviation industry began to develop a series of pre-flight checklists and inspection protocols that ultimately made the entire industry safer. These protocols focused on doing the same things the same way every time and were a big part of the safety improvements in the industry.

Over the last 20 years, the medical field has taken note of the success of the pre-flight checklists. Procedures and attention to detail have been incorporated in healthcare in a similar way through protocols and time-outs. Implementation of structured care is important in reducing errors and improving patient outcomes – the pediatric ICU (PICU) where I work is no exception.

The environment of the PICU, though too rigid for some, was where I thrived. Things that frustrated others — extensive and sometimes tedious charting, ever-changing patient care standards, and the frightening lability of PICU patients — were my comfort zone. I had tackled charge, resource, and preceptor roles faithfully in my home PICU. I had navigated the waters of the clinical and management track. I had negotiated with senior management teams, compromised with a variety of senior nursing staff, and nurtured newer nursing staff. I was a mega-advocate for my patients, my fellow PICU nurses, and, at times, for my profession.

The good, the bad, and the in-between. I had done it all.

But the monotony of it all was wearing. At least with aviation, once the safety checklist is done, you take off and get a change of scenery. In the PICU, once we had dotted our i's and crossed our t's, the outcomes were often the same: patient death and staff burnout. I had to keep reminding myself that sick and dying children are not normal days at work.

Around that time, I had a nursing friend tell me how transformative it was to do global health work. As cliché as her feelings about global health work sounded, I needed this inspiration. After being a nurse in the PICU for many years, I was dealing with serious compassion fatigue and secondary trauma.

Still, I must admit that I wasn't sure that mission work would be the answer. I had been on one medical mission in the past, and I was not convinced that it was for me. Why would another trip be different? How could I make sure that it was different?

As I considered doing another mission, I wondered what criteria would be important to a successful mission, so I began to do my research. Research does not always guarantee that you will be on a safe and successful mission, but it helps to eliminate some of the variables – lack of delegation, lack of organization, lack of skilled volunteers, lack of safety - that could cause a mission to fail. The organization that I had become so accustomed to in the PICU was key in my search.

Checklists and attention to detail were deeply important.

Soon it became evident to me that I wanted to work with an organization that addressed all of the aforementioned issues and believed in taking something small and broken and make it bigger and whole.

I ultimately found twelve organizations that I was willing to work with, so I applied and I waited. With little to no mission experience, it is always a little nerve-wracking when you apply. You never know who will accept you or what the out-of-pocket expenses may be. It can vary so much from organization to organization.

Ultimately, I chose to travel to Honduras with a group called Aloha Medical Missions that did cleft lip and other specialty surgeries along with dental work. The group was well-organized and included many return volunteers. Budgets and overhead were low, meaning that most of the money went into patient care in one form or another. Roles were preassigned prior to the mission based on individual skill sets. Most importantly, their communication was impeccable. As a PICU nurse, I understood that the attention given to pre-mission organization was critical to quality patient care.

After committing to this trip, I realized that not only did I know little about Honduras, but I had never considered traveling to Central America.

Here is what I did know – at the time, Honduras had one of the highest murder rates in the world. Many of its people were impoverished. It had one major highway dubiously called the Ronald Reagan Highway, likely because of the US military's efforts, some would say meddling, during the 1980's. This was done to win the hearts and minds of the Honduran people, not to mention to sway the simultaneous civil wars of Central America, in a way that served the best interest of the US.

In order to get to our home base in Comayagua, some fifty miles northwest of the capital, we had to fly into the Toncontin International Airport in Tegucigalpa. Flight professionals describe the airport's approach and landing as "a nightmare." The extremely short runway, the region's mountains, and the unusual maneuvers pilots must take to avoid them are no joke. When I learned this a day before I left, I figured this danger was apropos considering the responsibilities I had agreed to on this medical mission trip. I decided that the best course of action was to take adequate motion sickness medicine and pray for a safe landing, hoping that the safety protocols worked for both the flight and the mission.

Well, luck was upon me and the pre-flight checklists worked; we landed just fine in a country of which I had no knowledge.

What I hadn't prepared for was the winding, torturously long bus ride to Comayagua. The scenery of the countryside is romantic, but for those with motion sickness, it is daunting. The only pleasantry I found was in the 'hutch' middle fold out seat that was, ironically, the least claustrophobic. NOTE TO SELF: Always take the hutch seat in a bus.

When we finally arrived in Comayagua, I was assigned to an energetic team of health care professionals in the operating room that we affectionately dubbed the 'Aloha Room Four'. I should mention that while we agreed to our roles prior to leaving, this trip would include working with mostly adult patients and doing gynecology and specialized surgeries of the ears, nose, and throat.

A small portion of this trip would also include fitting patients for prosthetic limbs.

While I am a well-seasoned, headstrong, clinically competent PICU nurse, I only do pediatrics. No adults. No primary care. No artificial limb experience. No operating room experience.

I began to question what had I gotten myself into by agreeing to be a scrub nurse in the operating room for adult and pediatric ear, nose, and throat cases. I wondered if I was as flexible a nurse as I thought I was. Was I agreeing to something that I was not capable of carrying out? How would I make sense of all this on the first day of cases? Were the trip leaders going to see the shadow of a doubt that I had felt going into this?

I began to wonder — what was I getting myself into?

This is where organization and attention to detail came into play. In Comayagua, we found many similarities with hospitals in the United States. We adopted the same rituals of checking our emergency equipment, doing a full screening process, collaborating between health care professionals of potential patients, and performing a proper 'time out' (a safety checklist of sorts) once the patient was all set for their procedure or operation.

There were still vast differences. Most of the emergency equipment pieces had been used, and the screening process was laden with issues: language barriers, inaccurate histories, and absolutely no imaging capabilities, mind you. We were fortunate that we had a group of priests and local volunteers who carried us through some rough times when extra help was needed.

As for the other volunteers, Dr. Ron, our ear, nose, and throat surgeon, had the utmost confidence in my ability to take direction, which was important considering that I had very little practical experience with the instruments. His stories of being a physician in San Francisco during the AIDS epidemic have stayed with me. Dr. Jim from Hawaii, our faithful anesthesiologist, had a plethora of specialized practice and many medical missions under his belt. His leadership was evident in the operating room as we churned and burned our days. His experience teaching residents and fellows through the years showed. Laurie, from Virginia, was a carefree, spirited, and seasoned traveling nurse. Having her as the circulating nurse allowed the room to run smoothly, as she keenly anticipated what was needed at each next step. Her passion for travel, wonder, and positive outlook are why I am friends with her to this day. While it all felt like luck, it was actually a well-orchestrated symphony conducted by Dr. Margie Fine, a surgeon and the team leader of this trip, and her husband, Art Fine. Dr. Fine is one of the most seasoned and oldest female general surgeons in the country, and her husband is a skilled patent attorney. Not only were they our leaders, but both left us all with a sense of parental guidance that we needed on this trip.

Under Dr. Fine's level-headed leadership, Aloha Room Four thrived - and as Aloha Room Four thrived, so did I.

The stories of the people I met have stayed with me.

I met a local recovery room nurse who had many children. She discovered that we were the same age and practiced the same religion, but she was shocked to find that I am unmarried and without children.

Our housekeeper's daughter had a tonsillectomy and adenoidectomy while her mother worked tirelessly (and as a volunteer) for the entire week. But cleaning was everyone's job, and it was not unusual to find the highly esteemed OBGYN physician with a mop in hand, cleaning his room.

We all checked our egos at the door and did what needed to be done.

Our evenings and downtime were equally fulfilling. Our conversation revolved around philanthropy, volunteering, religion, and politics. Health care work is often a thankless job, but the pride that I felt when our team leaders recognized each of us individually for our sacrifices that week was refreshing. There was plenty of fun, cheap beer, bland food, and simple provisions. I had the most mouthwatering plantains in this world and waited anxiously to eat them at every meal (and I don't even like bananas).

Of course, traveling in a developing country presents challenges that you don't often experience at home. In many countries, infrastructure and sanitation services are difficult to find. I remember all the litter that overwhelmed my sense of smell. The safety of the team is an important obligation for the organization. For our protection, there were armed guards with us at all times, even when we left the hotel or hospital. During the heart of the mission, there was no downtime to process the day-to-day activities, nor to develop a coping plan to mask the horror of poverty and filth that I saw. But the support of the team that week was enough to keep me moving forward.

Then, there were the physical challenges of traveling on poorly maintained roads in older vehicles. We got the two flat tires that nearly derailed us from our fun team-building activities. We were on the way to a gorgeous national park where we hiked to a waterfall in the rain, wearing trash bags to ward of the elements. These things are all part of the experience when working in different parts of the world.

Honduras surprised me.

There were the crafts of artisans handed down through the generations, majestic mountain ranges whose names I cannot even recall, painted advertisements on the walls, and the Comayagua Cathedral that houses the oldest clock in the Americas. Sometimes, when I close my eyes, I can still envision the view from the top of the Cathedral, a black bird soaring overhead.

Then, there was the work that we were there to do. Many patients came to the operating room with rosaries in hand. We could barely communicate, yet a simple touch of the hand or smile eased their fears.

Even though I never thought of Central America as a place that I was interested in, my time in Honduras made it so worthwhile.

Good medical mission trip leaders can give a trip meaning, and local support is imperative. A cohesive team will always surpass a solo performance. This success never fails to astonish me. In the United States, I was always confident that we could make magic, but I was not always as confident overseas.

In the beginning, this medical mission trip was shrouded in uncertainties and dangers. What came out of it was an experience that allowed me to flourish both personally and professionally. I felt rejuvenated after the trip. The other volunteers inspired me just as much as the patients and the families did. I proved my worth by displaying my flexibility, confidence, and passion which I continue to carry with me on every new trip because of Honduras.

The greatest lesson that I have learned from my time in Honduras is that if stretch yourself outside of your comfort zone and trust in others, good things can happen. You will rise to the challenge and succeed based on your clinical skills, knowledge, judgement calls, trust in others, and longevity in the field of nursing.

The truth is that magic happens. It happens because of good planning and organization – the pre-flight checklist, as it were. Missions around the world accomplish what we were able to do in Comayagua: provide care for people and renew my purpose as a nurse.

Do No Harm
Amanda Judd

The evening sun set over the misty East African mountainside as we snaked up the red-earth road past small villages to our compound. This was our home base for the first week of the mission. We were much higher up on the mountain than indicated in our itinerary, but maybe this was part of the adventure.

After a brief dinner, the team gathered to empty the medical bags. We stood shivering on the cold sidewalk in our ill-planned clothing that had been packed for the intense heat of the East African savannah. Our crystalline breaths made vapor puffs as we pulled out the duffels. A chilling damp soaked our bones as we stood emptying the packs of their belongings.

Some duffels were filled with stuffed animals. *An interesting choice for a medical clinic*, I thought. Other bags held used braces and sunglasses, slightly more useful, but still not the critical medicine that we needed. When we finally came across the medication bags, we found many medicines that were expired and useless, and a very limited supply of those medications that *were* useful.

I mentioned to the team leader that we barely had enough medications for two clinics of the six clinics that we had planned. I wondered aloud about who had prepared these bags. Clearly, it was someone who didn't understand the importance of essential medicines that are the gold standard used in humanitarian aid work — medications specifically selected for relevance and cost-efficacy.

My heart sank. I worried for the patients' safety. Prescribing the wrong medications could have adverse effects on patients and even cause death. I became acutely aware of the importance of utilizing the knowledge of the one doctor on the trip.

I collapsed into bed that night hoping that the clinics were more organized than our medical bags and team.

Our first clinic day started with the usual set-up of the pharmacy, triage, and patient rooms for the crowd waiting outside. We had a large group of non-medical volunteers along with small medical team of two nurses and one doctor, who we soon discovered was only staying for half of the trip. I became very concerned because not only did we have the wrong medications, but with the doctor leaving early, we had limited medical guidance.

Soon, we sat down to see patients and asked for our translator. As it turned out, we had a succession of three translators. The first was a lab worker who left because he had work to do, the second a local nurse who refused to directly translate and instead said things like, "They have arthritis and a cough for two days. They need antibiotics." Our last translator was a lovely gentleman with a generous smile dressed in a military uniform. As the long day wound down, we thanked him for his help. He stood and turned to us, asking, "May I be seen now?"

We were shocked to discover that our organization had not hired translators. They had pulled this man from the crowd while he was waiting to be seen and made him translate for the day. This seriously jeopardized patient privacy, especially since he was from the community. I felt terrible about him having to work to be treated.

We quickly assessed him and then ushered him over to the pharmacy where we found our team leader — who was in charge of the pharmacy — upset. Evidently, one of the local hospital workers had come in and pilfered about half of our two-day supply of medications. The team leader had done nothing to stop him. Crowd control was nonexistent and perhaps with the masses bearing down she felt overwhelmed, but it was never made clear to us why this theft had been allowed; all we knew was that it had to stop if we were to have even part of the medications that we would need for the remaining clinics.

On missions, unexpected things will happen, but having structured clinics with a planned formulary, an organized flow of patients, and official translators should be the standard for any medical humanitarian work. Properly planned missions should not operate in chaos; even organizations that work in the most dangerous conflict zones have structure and protocols. This suddenly felt less like a medical mission and more like some sort of misguided cultural tour.

I was unsure that we had done any good in that village, but a local minister said, "The fact that you are here changes people's perception that there are people who care. Drinkers will stop drinking for the day, so it is an effect that will be felt over time."

I felt that statement was optimistic at best.

The days that followed were more of the same, chaos served with a side of not enough medication or medical staff.

Our patients were quite ill and in desperate need of competent care and follow-up. Severe hypertension and diabetes were common. Deadly typhoid was raging through some of the communities. Brucella was rampant from the unpasteurized milk that everyone drank. Cases of Pott's Disease and other extra-pulmonary tuberculosis (TB) were frequent, not to mention the ambiguous cases of night sweats and weight loss – a common sign of HIV, which we were unable to test for.

We had to treat pulmonary TB positive patients; yet we had no respirators to protect ourselves from contracting the life-threatening airborne infection.

With the illness burden high and the number of patients endless, it was abundantly clear that we lacked enough medical staff to run a clinic, so within a few days, the in-country sponsors brought in local clinical officers to help. Clinical officers are the equivalent of a nurse practitioner or physician assistant. They held a wealth of knowledge about local health issues and conditions and became invaluable to us.

I was grateful for the clinical officers and wondered if they were aware of the mission's incompetence — how could they not be? Either way, without a physician present, we became deeply dependent on the clinical officers to the point that our presence was unnecessary, a dog and pony show with our inept team from the US bringing the patients in while the national staff did all of the work.

My mind kept wandering to the words of Jan Egeland, former UN Undersecretary for Humanitarian Affairs: "Saving human lives is no place for amateurs. Why is that? Because the poor, dispossessed, and disaster-prone should have at least one basic right left to them: to be protected from incompetence."[1]

We changed clinic sites daily, and the last clinic day was no different. We had left the mountainside for the scorched earth of the savannah. The clinic site in the wooden church was dark and dusty with very little light streaming through the slats. The hot air was suffocating. The woman was one of the first through the door. Her dry, loose skin belied her age of thirty, and she listed to the side as she walked up to the table. Her clothes hung off of her as if she were little girl in her mother's rags. She was emaciated, with a gaunt face and desperate eyes.

She had come for one thing: "I am here for the HIV vaccine. The man on the radio said that you have the vaccine."

My God, what exactly are we doing? There is no HIV vaccine. Who would be so awful as to announce this on the radio? Our team's disorganization felt more than negligent and unethical — it felt cruel.

I had betrayed everything that my gut told me not to do on this mission, and it put me in situations that compromised my ethics and my care. These thoughts were so pervasive that I began to have a real crisis of conscience. Humanitarian work was something that I strongly believed in, and yet we were so unequipped to help at all. The term "moral distress" kept coming up in our conversations about the indifference of the recently departed American doctor and the lack of caregivers and appropriate medications. As a nurse, I struggled with the position we were in.

Watching that woman walk out of the building, her body sagging with grief and the loss of her last breath of hope, haunts me to this day.

As we sat in the crowded airport waiting to go home, our flight was delayed. I was reeling with confusion, questioning whether I should ever do global health work again.

Just then, I received word from one of the people that we met on the mission. He said that the store near our hotel, which my team had frequented during our stay, had been bombed right after we left. The violence was a gutting reminder of the desperate situation that the people living in developing nations and areas of conflict face all too often. This was one of the many reasons that I was originally compelled to do humanitarian work, to help the underserved and those who through no fault of their own could not access care. This was my final and lasting impression of the country.

I looked out from the small airplane window over the dusty savannah as the forbidding sky sat gloaming over the cradle of humanity. Desperately anticipating my next breaths of more familiar air, I struggled, reflecting on the many ways that my decisions had betrayed my own instincts, and as time went on I came to the bitter realization that the carelessness of this humanitarian work was not an indictment of a place or culture. Rather it was a judgment on us, the team. The failures of this mission were the result of the lack of formal medical planning, leadership, and education needed to execute a successful mission. It was arrogance, pure and simple.

I resolved that if I was ever to do this work again, I must demand a standard of ethics and care because without one, we may do more harm than good.

Reference list:

1. Heintze H-J, Thielbörger P. *International Humanitarian Action: NOHA Textbook*. Cham: Springer; 2018.

The Humanitarian Roundtable: What We Want You to Know

We thought it was important to include a virtual roundtable of interviews about what humanitarian workers thought was important. The responses below are from novice to expert medical volunteers and national staff. Thank you to Elise Peterson, Monserrat Dieguez, Kasey Hostetler, and other interviewees who chose to remain anonymous.

In general, what is the national staff's perception of expats coming to volunteer in your country/community?

- There is a combination of gratitude and expectation of all the amazing things that we are going to witness, as well as what we will learn in the process.

If you could give advice to an expat starting to work with you, what would it be? How to fit in, what attitude to adopt, how to work well with local people, how to be most effective in the time they will be there, etc.

- Be flexible, in all situations. Take your direction from the local needs. A thorough assessment, implementation, and evaluation is key.

- There is a lot of misinformation when it comes to health in the underserved communities, so education of the community is as important as medicine. (Health knowledge amongst women is typically lower.) Because of the lack of access to healthcare, there is a lot of self-medication. I have witnessed the positive response that people have when a healthcare provider thoroughly explains a diagnosis, medications, etc. And, never forget to smile.

- Adaptability and an open mind are essential attitudes to have before entering any kind of humanitarian work. Usually these traits are inherent in any health care/humanitarian worker, but I think it's important to do a self-check prior to starting your work and to proactively take down any mental barriers or biases you might have before going on a mission.

Does the national staff ever feel like we make your job more difficult?

- Sometimes, but it really does depend on the individual who you are working with. I personally have had difficulties with students because it seems they are so focused on getting everything right and making sure they are making the correct questions that the human touch gets lost somewhere along the way.

What misconceptions do expats have about the local staff and facilities?

- I know there are rural areas that don't provide many accommodations and therefore some of the locals may confuse being impoverished with poor personal hygiene. (I believe that happens everywhere.) However, there have been some unkind comments I have heard about it.

What positive or negative impact do humanitarian workers leave in the community? If negative, what should you do to prevent this?

- Positives are teaching and educating local staff in the home countries because they will remain caring for the population when we go home.
- Negative aspects are lack of planning prior to trip, non-medical people in trip leadership positions [making medical decisions that they are not qualified to make], and pacifying the locals based on their expectations.
- I definitely see many more positive impacts than negative. A negative impact that I have seen are that sometimes locals will bring candy, fruit, etc. as a token of their appreciation and have it rejected. It's totally okay if you won't eat it, but at least take it.
- Things that negatively impact the community are traveling in posh cars, disregarding the poverty level of

the community, or eating canned food and disposing the can near a community that is struggling to eat.

What do local communities think of external organizations and individual volunteers?

- Communities are more accepting of an external organization as opposed to care coming from the government. [Here] it's because most of the time there is a political party involved with governmental care.

What is it like in a community when the organization leaves? For the population? For the workers?

- For the population, I would say relief, a sense of hope that their illness has been taken care of. For me as a translator, it is very rewarding. I am able to help the ones that came to help and help the ones looking for help. It's fuel for the soul.
- When a humanitarian project closes, the national staff are affected first in terms of losing their jobs. The community is affected because they quickly adapt to their old ways.

Have you had a particularly difficult experience with a person or organization? What particular behaviors/attitudes/ viewpoints lead to these issues?

- It was with a particular person. It was a NP student getting her Master's. She did not show any emotion to the patients and did not speak to me, except to translate. It was very a difficult and uncomfortable situation. I wondered how she treated patients back home.

What is your most memorable experience, positive or negative, with an expat or organization?

- At the organization that I have worked with there is always a devotional at the beginning of the day. That morning I decided to speak and explain how much of an impact the work had, not just to one person but how it impacted the whole community. It turns out that there were lot of conflicts with the mission's OR staff and they had decided just to call off the surgeries for the week and have only clinic running. (I was not aware of this when I gave my devotional.) When I shared, the OR staff remembered why they were there. They decided to put their differences aside and continue doing the surgeries.
- Having a cultural component built into our everyday experience to learn about the people in the region better allowed us to care for the Indian people during clinic.

- The people I met, both local and foreign, while working there have left a lasting impression on me. Their knowledge, humility, and strength all impressed me to my core.
- People! I have made friends for life on almost every trip I have taken, either other team members or locals.

If you could sit down and talk to an expat who is going to go to your country/community to volunteer, what advice would you give him or her? Please be as specific and extensive as you can.

- America is a continent, not a country.
- Open your mind. What you are about to see and experience will have an amazing impact that will mark your life forever.
- Talk to family or friends that might have been in that country before, even as tourists. Google, read as much as you can about it. Don't make assumptions. (I once heard that someone was very surprised we had malls in my country!)
- Flexibility—nothing is beneath you—surgeon mopping the floor, nurse running the code. Kindness—a smile goes a long way. Forgiveness—other cultures and countries do not know your experience and we do not know theirs—be forgiving of ignorance.

How does a population view expats coming for a short time?

- Well, it depends. If they are medical providers or any type of program like house building, education etc., there is a great sense of gratitude for the help that is being given. I would say locals would like to have people to stay for longer periods of time. However, in my country, due to the civil war, anything that has to do with military creates a lot of fear and mistrust.

- Our first perception of expatriates is that they are bringing jobs. We know for sure that they cannot do whatever they have come to do without involving the locals. In the process of working we will learn new things and also make friends.

How does the local population think of medicines - pills versus shots vs no pill/shot but rather exercise, diet, massage, etc?

- I don't know if it's something lacking in the general education, but I have witnessed that people would rather get pills or even request surgeries. When they are told it is not necessary, they feel somewhat upset.

How does the population view traditional healers? Traditional birth attendants?

- In the Mayan culture, it's very common to see natural medicine. It's something that has been passed on from generation to generation. Mostly in the rural areas, women feel more confident in midwives than going to a hospital. Very sadly, I will say that is because of how much racism there is towards indigenous people and woman, not to mention the language barrier from Spanish to the Mayan languages.

- Very favorably. Of course, I believe in the practice of western medicine, but enough cannot be said about the positive impact traditional healers have on their patients who believe so strongly in them.

In reference to patients and coworkers, are there things we should never do? Always do?

- Always try, as much as the circumstances permit it, to keep a positive state of mind.
- Always be flexible.
- Being intimate in public is a no-no.
- When an expat gets romantic with a national staff, it may affect the work place negatively depending on the character of the national staff. One female staff member influenced an expat to hate me for no clear reason which almost cost me my job.
- Another bit of advice that I would like to give is about the dress code. Here in Northern Uganda, mini-skirts are always seen as the dress of non-serious people.
- A national staff worker will feel betrayed if he/she learns that the expat supervisor is less knowledgeable than him/her on that particular field of work.

Do expats ask questions or have all the answers? Do they expect to learn from us or share with us?

- I would definitely think that it is a learning process on both sides; therefore, communication is always key to making the whole experience as smooth as possible.

How are women viewed within your country and what is their role? Are women talked down to?

- Yes, especially in rural areas. Although most of the time woman's role is as the provider of income, food, and labor, they are still talked down. In spite of this oppression, many women have been inspired to help their community grow. They have found the courage to truly make a difference.

What if expats don't speak the language? Does a translator say word for word what we say or adapt it to the context for understanding?

- Personally, I will explain the word to the expat that I am working with the simplest terms that can be used, so that way we can make the translation as accurate as possible.
- Speaking in first person and asking for clarification is always important.

As a healthcare worker, do you spend time at home exploring medical issues that you will deal with, educating yourself on global health, and taking classes on global health before you are in-country?

- I personally did not, but I was working under my EMT license and was in full-time nursing school, so I just didn't have much time to. Plus, I was fortunate enough to work under/with a team of experienced ER doctors and a paramedic and did most of my learning on the spot from them.
- I am biased as I took many courses in global health during my MPH degree which were incredibly helpful.
- Yes!

Do you actively look for a mission organization with strong medical leadership practicing in areas where the patients will have access to follow-up after you leave? Does your organization work on local staff education? Is this important to you?

- Yes. I went to Bernard Mevs hospital in Haiti because I understood that their program worked in a partnership with local students and professionals to promote learning and experience, with an end goal being local independence and long term sustainability for the hospital. The overseas volunteers were a smaller, but still important, part of the big pie. Local staff education was huge and there were many training programs in effect while I was serving there, often happening independent of the main flow of the hospital. We also worked side-by-side with nursing students, local EMTs (who were often our best resources and interpreters), and under local doctors.

- Absolutely. Our foundation prides itself on setting up "MASH Units". While they are helpful in certain situations, we strive to educate and help develop a self-sustaining solution.

If you do not speak the language, do you verify that the organization has hired translators?

- Yes, always.
- That seems like it would be a necessary hurdle to overcome in some way. The organization I had was all set up with local translators, so I didn't put too much thought into it.

How do you feel about photographing patients?

- This is fine, but only with consent.
- I've seen incredibly powerful photos of patients on social media, and the emotions those photos stir up in me are ones of empathy that motivate me to be proactive about seeking out experiences to help others like them. In the moment, however, I do feel slightly ashamed about taking photos of patients and usually don't.
- All good as long as they approve.

- Taking photos also needs consent to make it a positive impact. There is a wide belief that expats get lots of money from the photos they take, especially photos of needy people.

Anything else you would like to add so we can bring all these ideas to people wishing to volunteer abroad?

- Always vet your organization fully.
- There is no small role in volunteering. Martin Luther King once said, "Life's most urgent question is what are we doing for others."

Trust your gut
Emily Scott

My last good day in Sierra Leone was a Tuesday, the day before I found out that one of my colleagues had Ebola.

It was my first day off since arriving in-country, and I had plans to meet some friends from my Partners In Health (PIH) team at the beach. After spending a few days together at Maforki Ebola Treatment Unit, caring for patients in the Red Zone, the twelve of us had been split up to work at different facilities based on where Partners In Health leadership thought we would be most useful. Most of my cohort had remained in the Port Loko district to either continue working at Maforki or to help out at the Government Hospital where patients with non-Ebola-related health issues were treated.

While it may seem like Government Hospital would be an ideal place to work because you wouldn't have to worry about Ebola, in reality many of us felt that working there was more dangerous than suiting up at Maforki each day. In an Ebola Treatment Unit, at least we knew where we stood: Our patients had the deadly disease, and each time we interacted with them, we had to take the proper precautions to protect ourselves. Government Hospital was more of a gray area. No patients with Ebola were expected to enter the facility, so clinicians did not need to don their full Personal Protective Equipment (PPE) when entering the wards. If you're treating a patient for cancer or malaria, there's no need to wear a hazmat suit to do it.

But what if a patient with Ebola slipped through the imperfect triage system at Government Hospital and was admitted to the ward under the assumption that they were suffering from a different disease? Or what if someone was admitted while incubating the virus but before becoming symptomatic? Ebola has a 21-day incubation period, meaning that if I contracted the virus, I could walk around for up to three weeks without showing symptoms and without being contagious. I wondered how often the Government Hospital re-screened its patients after admission. If a patient was admitted with malaria and a few days later started showing symptoms of Ebola, would someone notice in time to protect the clinicians who had been treating him without full PPE?

I never worked at Government Hospital, so I really can't say for sure. I have heard varying opinions from the doctors and nurses who served there: some say they felt perfectly safe, and others say that they had serious concerns from their first shift. Our colleague who contracted Ebola first collapsed at Government Hospital, but he had also worked with the rest of us at Maforki days earlier. It's anyone's guess where and how he became exposed to Ebola.

I never saw Government Hospital myself because I was sent back to the capital, Freetown, to work at Princess Christian

Maternity Hospital, the Ebola Holding Center for pregnant women. By the time I arrived, local doctors and nurses knew that delivering a baby from an Ebola-positive mother was likely a death sentence for the caregiver. There are so many fluids with such high viral loads involved in a delivery that it was incredibly risky to give any medical care to a laboring woman if she had Ebola. They also knew that Ebola-infected pregnant women were likely to die anyway; rather than give them preferential treatment, healthcare workers focused on the patients they thought they could save. Unfortunately for West African women, labor and delivery looks frighteningly like Ebola. Even normal labor shares many symptoms with the deadly virus: abdominal pain, nausea, headache, weakness, bleeding. Complications of labor that look like Ebola, such as fever or seizures, were common in Sierra Leone because health systems were abysmal even before the outbreak. The end result was that obstetric care essentially ceased in Sierra Leone. The only maternity hospital in the country became a ghost town. Women wandered the halls carrying the babies they had lost when no medical professionals would come to care for them. Laboring women, whether they actually had Ebola or not, were on their own.

In response to this disaster, a Holding Center was set up in front of the maternity hospital to screen pregnant women for Ebola. In a small cement building that had previously been used for radiology, staff wearing full protective suits tested and cared for laboring women. The screening process required two negative blood tests 72 hours apart before the women could be allowed to enter the full maternity hospital for obstetric care.

That was longer than many women could wait for life-saving treatment.

Despite the horrors my patients faced, I woke up each day excited to share my skills as a labor and delivery nurse. I noticed imperfections in infection prevention and control policies in our unit from day one. Personal protective equipment was not standardized; a lack of staff meant that sometimes we had to doff our suits without a spotter watching us; I knew of coworkers who felt ill but shrugged it off or treated themselves at home instead of reporting their symptoms to leadership. I did my best to protect myself while I worked with my colleagues to address the safety issues. While I wished my concerns had been taken more seriously, my desire to continue my work completely outweighed the level of risk I felt I was taking.

When my day off coincided with that of some good friends who worked hours away at Maforki, I jumped at the chance to meet them at the beach to decompress and share our experiences. We had a fantastic day of swimming in the surf, sunning ourselves on the beach, and unloading difficult stories of our work over a healing beer or two. It was jarring to think that a short drive away from the peaceful turquoise surf, people were fighting a deadly disease in horrific conditions. But we put Ebola aside for the day and lingered as long as we could while the sun sank lower and lower toward the water.

Among the news my friend shared with me that day was the fact that one of our colleagues had collapsed while working at Government Hospital. Several other clinicians came immediately to his aid, assuming that he had fainted from heat exhaustion. Sierra Leone is very hot, and clinicians were working very hard; it didn't surprise me to hear that one of us had passed out from the effort. If you're used to working in an air-conditioned hospital with plenty of staff, it is a shock to run from one emergency to the next in a poorly-ventilated ward in 90-degree heat. I told my friend to give our colleague a hug and a stern talking-to about taking better care of himself. I did not feel that we had any reason to worry about him.

I was still in my pajamas the next morning when a PIH staff member knocked on my door and asked me to come downstairs for a meeting. Again, I thought nothing of it. All of the staff assembled in our common area, unconcerned and chatting away. A high-level member of PIH leadership that I hadn't met materialized, and I wondered what was important enough to get us all out of bed to meet with a man who certainly had more important things to do. He told the group that in four months of working in West Africa, PIH had never had a clinician become infected with Ebola. Suddenly, I realized what was coming. As the weight of it settled heavy on my shoulders, I knew what he was going to say before he said it. Our colleague had tested positive for Ebola.

I struggled to process the news because most of my friends were hours away in Port Loko. Almost everyone else in Freetown was from a cohort that had just arrived in-country, and I was one of only a few people who knew the infected clinician. As far as I was concerned, there was only one thing to do at that moment: I went back upstairs, put on my scrubs, and went to the Holding Unit to care for my patients. I donned my PPE and entered the Red Zone, trying to focus on the task at hand rather than the questions swirling through my head.

Shortly after our American colleague fell ill, one of PIH's Sierra Leonean clinicians was also confirmed to have Ebola. Suddenly, PIH clinicians began reporting cases of diarrhea or fever that they had been ignoring. Everyone had a different theory for how our friends had been exposed. We replayed everything in our minds: who had we hugged in the last few days? Who had we shaken hands with? We began to regret our relaxed standards for physical contact.

Within a week, sixteen American PIH staffers were sent home on chartered flights after the Centers for Disease Control deemed them "high risk" for having physical contact with the infected clinicians after they became symptomatic. The Maforki Ebola Treatment Unit was permanently closed due to safety deficiencies. It was a frightening few days, with the ever-present question pressing at the back of my mind: "Am I next?" I was certain that my American colleague had followed safety procedures exactly, just as I felt I had. Where was the breach that had exposed him? Had he and the Sierra Leonean clinician made the same mistake without realizing it? Had I?

PIH leadership and the World Health Organization carried out an investigation into infection prevention and control procedures at PIH facilities. My colleagues and I stepped forward with issues and suggestions while we waited to see what the next step would be. After a few days, several members of my cohort and I reluctantly decided that it was no longer safe to continue our work in Sierra Leone.

It was an incredibly difficult decision. I can say with certainty that absolutely no one I worked with *wanted* to leave - least of all me. I felt that the work we were doing at the maternity hospital was important, and I honestly wish I could still be there. In dark moments, I think about the women I could have helped if I had stayed longer, and I hope I didn't abandon someone to die because I wanted to protect myself. I continue to be confident in my decision, although it broke my heart to walk away.

I don't doubt the good intentions of Partners In Health. They leapt into the fray in West Africa during the peak of the outbreak when they certainly didn't have to. The first teams of PIH clinicians bravely provided care at Maforki when the unit held 100 patients in absolutely horrific conditions. Having been there when we had only 10 patients, I am in awe of those teams. I admire those clinicians' courage and the risks they took in the service of those who needed it most.

But could processes have been done better, made safer, and the level of care improved between those first days and the last? I think so. The events during and after our colleague's fight against Ebola have shed light on those issues, and on what changes need to be made.

I am hopeful that PIH has been addressing infection prevention and control issues and improving the safety of their clinicians while continuing their commitment to the people of West Africa. By their own admission, emergency response isn't PIH's specialty; they are an organization that normally works on long-term development projects. With the outbreak officially long over, PIH's real area of expertise is what's needed — health system strengthening. After the last case of Ebola was gone and the emergency response groups had left, PIH has committed to remaining in Sierra Leone and Liberia for years. They will continue to work in government hospitals and to rebuild the ineffective health systems that the outbreak destroyed.

Shortly after I left, I heard that another facility in which PIH works had received its first case of measles. With vaccination programs shut down for nearly a year during the Ebola crisis, West Africa was a measles outbreak waiting to happen. Care of pregnant women and newborns was abysmal before Ebola, and even worse after. Common illnesses like malaria, typhoid, cancer, heart disease… you name it, and I guarantee you wouldn't want to be treated in Sierra Leone if you came down with it. PIH stayed in West Africa to try to change that. Years after the outbreak has ended, PIH is still in working in Sierra Leone today. They have set up an eye care program for survivors because complications of Ebola can lead to blindness. They continue to treat patients in hospitals and clinics for everyday issues like malaria, malnutrition, and pregnancy. They are also working to remodel health facilities in order to make them safer and more effective for both patients and caregivers.

Our American and Sierra Leonean colleagues who caught Ebola survived, and no other PIH clinicians contracted the disease. After arriving home from Sierra Leone, I spent three weeks off work waiting out my incubation period – 21 days from my last shift in the Red Zone. I had plenty of time to think about my experiences and share them with the rest of my cohort, who were also checking their temperatures twice a day and counting down their monitoring periods. Some blamed PIH, while others vehemently defended them. We felt anger, disappointment, regret, but also pride in our work and confidence that we had done the right thing. I find some truth in all of these responses. Very little in global health is ever completely black and white.

There are a hundred different lessons I could take away from my time in Sierra Leone, but the one that sticks with me is trust your gut. If you worry for the safety of yourself and your team, speak up. For those of us who travel to far-flung places to help those the world has forgotten, putting ourselves first can seem anathema, but you cannot take care of others if you aren't taking care of yourself. Now, when I board planes on the way to my next medical mission, I listen carefully as the flight attendant reminds me to put on my oxygen mask on first before assisting others.

Sierra Leone also taught me something priceless about myself: I'm not going to stop. Ebola response was hard in ways that I didn't anticipate, but I do not regret going. I'm going to experience events that terrify me and situations that are out of my control, but that sure as hell doesn't mean I'm going to stay home. I get to use this experience to make my next mission better and safer, to understand my response to the unexpected, to prepare myself more fully. I will not stop doing this work, but I *will* ask more of the organizations with which I serve.

I see every mission as a building block. I'm not perfect, and neither is any organization that I will serve with, but I get a little closer to it every time I deploy somewhere that asks for my help. I want to be the best humanitarian nurse that I am capable of being, and that means challenging myself, learning from mistakes, and bringing that knowledge into my next mission. I can't wait to get going.

The Suffering Grass:
The Nurse as Witness
Amanda Judd

Silence equals complicity.

A Kikuyu proverb: "*When elephants fight, it is the grass that suffers.*"
In Swahili, "Wapiganapo tembo nyasi huumia."

At what point does the silence of a nurse on a humanitarian medical mission imply complicity? It's a question I ask myself every time I return from such a mission and write about the work, carefully choosing my words to protect the privacy of women who are victims of violence and rape.

I've consciously refrained from speaking out on the subject in light of my own culture's xenophobia. Besides, although violence against women happens everywhere, the topic makes people terribly uncomfortable.

India

I was in India the first time I encountered what I'm referring to, and when I asked about it, was puzzled by what I was told. Women who came to the makeshift medical clinic were clearly upset, expressing their emotions in a litany of words I didn't understand. When I asked the translators what they said, the answer came in just one of two words—either "cough" or "dizziness."

I had a nagging feeling the translators were editing what was being said to keep me from fully comprehending what the women were communicating. Was it out of embarrassment or because of politeness? I will never know. Maybe it was nothing. Or were the women who came to the clinic and were so upset crying out for help?

When the mission was completed, I traveled throughout India sightseeing. Out in the hinterlands, far away from television and other media, I explored villages and visited the country's ancient stepwells, unaware of what had happened back in Delhi. By the time I arrived in Jaipur, the violent rape and subsequent death of Jyoti Singh had made headlines all over the world.[1] The event that had occurred was so unfathomable it was difficult to process. The graphic nature of the rape's news coverage left me feeling sick.

When I returned to Delhi a week after Jyoti's death, the city was completely transformed from the one I had visited earlier. Even the laws had changed. Violent protests wracked the city. Indians were angry and upset, and they vehemently condemned what had happened. The days of blame-the-victim mentality seemed numbered in India. Jyoti, known at the time only as India's Daughter, remained nameless due to the nation's laws. She deserved a voice—to be heard and not forgotten.

As I reflected on my work at the clinic, I again began to wonder what message my female patients had been trying to convey. Later, on a mission to East Africa, it became personal for me.

East Africa

I was in a cold, damp hospital room seeing patients when a confident woman with a young girl walked through the door. The woman was a teacher who spoke English, so the possibility of mistranslation wasn't an issue.

The girl, she explained, was a student about 9 years old who had been raped multiple times by her uncle. Sitting with the local clinical officer (similar to a nurse practitioner), I listened to the story while staring at a wall poster on how to medically and legally handle rape cases in that country.

The teacher said that the girl's mother—a prostitute—was unable to protect her. She was unwilling to act against the uncle who was violating the child. When the officer asked if there was any way to get the girl out of the situation, the teacher's response was heart-stopping.

"I would take the girl into *my* home," she said, "but I currently have two other female students living with me because they were being raped at home. I can't take in another student."

The officer's response was silence. Nothing could be done.

So there it was: the poster on the wall paying lip service to handling of rape juxtaposed with the reality of being powerless; of being female in a world where females are the most vulnerable of the vulnerable; of being female in a world of men—grass trampled by elephants.

Everywhere I've traveled, I've heard various versions of this same sad story: *It's normal as a woman to be beaten by your husband. It's the woman's fault. There's nothing to be done if you're raped.*

As the World Health Organization reports, being female is a liability but being poor and female can put a woman in dire circumstances.[2] Women are inherently at more risk than men.[3] Females living in poverty are the least likely group to get educated.[4] Women are less likely to have income, and when they do have income, there are gender disparities.[5] Women are less likely to have power to stand up to violence.[6]

The grass needs a voice

No absolute guidelines exist on how to deal with this; every situation is different. There is only one conclusion I come to when I reflect on my unwillingness to speak: Silence equals complicity. Complicity perpetuates trauma.

I invite other nurses to join me—not to exploit the suffering of others but to empower the powerless and victimized everywhere.

As professionals, nurses must be vocal in bearing witness. We can no longer be complicit in rape and violence against women around the world. We should no longer remain silent about the Jyotis of the world, girls raped and brutalized, and women who are beaten because men are expected to beat their wives. We cannot change a culture, but we can be a voice for the disempowered.

If we give the grass a voice, it does not have to suffer.

Reference list:

1. "India's Daughter." *PBS*, Public Broadcasting Service, www.pbs.org/independentlens/films/indias-daughter/.

2. "Violence against Women." *World Health Organization*, World Health Organization, 5 Feb. 2018, www.who.int/mediacentre/factsheets/fs239/en/.

3. Johnson, Kirsten. "Association of Sexual Violence and Human Rights Violations With Physical and Mental Health in Territories of the Eastern Democratic Republic of the Congo." *JAMA*, American Medical Association, 4 Aug. 2010, jamanetwork.com/journals/jama/fullarticle/186342.

4. UNESCO. "Gender Review: Creating Sustainable Futures for All." *Global Education Monitoring Report*, 2016, doi:http://unesdoc.unesco.org/images/0024/002460/246045e.pdf.

5. "Facts and Figures: Economic Empowerment." *UN Women*, www.unwomen.org/en/what-we-do/economic-empowerment/facts-and-figures.

6. Guimond, Marie-France, and Katie Robinette. "A Survivor behind Every Number: Using Programme Data on Violence against Women and Girls in the Democratic Republic of Congo to Influence Policy and Practice." *Taylor & Francis*, 26 June 2014, www.tandfonline.com/doi/full/10.1080/13552074.2014.9209 79?scroll=top&needAccess=true.

Originally published in Reflections on Nursing Leadership, Vol 43-3, May 25, 2017; ©2017 Sigma Theta Tau International, used with permission

Follow The Money

Sue Averill

Humanitarian Work: noble, selfless, kind. We forget that humanitarian work is performed in countries with great needs but also great pride. Every country in the world has medical systems in place, but in the "developing world" those systems are often minimally functional or corrupted. It is within those systems humanitarian work is performed. And sidetracked. And frequently thwarted.

We want to believe that our efforts will be received with the same noble kindness with which they are offered. However, in spite of our best efforts, greed and power oftentimes prevail.

While working as a nurse with *Médecins Sans Frontières* (*MSF*) in northern Uganda, I was asked to cover a three-week break for the physician of a stable, long-term Kala Azar (Leishmaniasis) project in Amudat District. Amudat sits on the eastern border that Uganda shares with Kenya. The dominant Karamajong tribe shares this mostly wild and undeveloped scrubland with the smaller Pokot tribe.

It's easy to recognize the difference by tribal dress.

Karamajong men wear stovepipe-style, multicolored hats perched atop their heads and plaid blankets tied across one shoulder. Women weave brightly colored beads into their dresses. The Pokot men wrap fabric around their waists in a skirt-like fashion. The women shave their heads except for one small tuft of hair braided with beads. They often pierce their lips with shells and safety pins.

For both tribes, cattle herding and hunting occupy the men. Men and boys once lived among their cattle with only a spear, bow and arrow, and blanket, but automatic rifles have changed that landscape. Ever since, cattle raiding has become a deadly sport.

The two tribes don't get along. In fact, "Pokot" means "Enemy" in the Karamajong language. Typically, a stronger tribe will dominate positions of power in local government services, such as jobs, education, and even health care. As the underdogs in any confrontation or distribution of supplies, the Pokot tribe usually came out drawing the short straw, even during disease outbreaks.

Just as I was receiving my handover briefing, reports of meningitis came from nearby government-run health units.

When you don't share a common language, determining the cause of an outbreak isn't always easy, but the best method of communication is often pantomime. In this situation, a Karamajong elder grabs the back of his neck, rolls his eyes upwards until only the whites show, and stiffens his entire body: a perfect description of meningitis.

In such a mobile society, diseases like meningitis can spread quickly. Uganda lies within a swath of Africa known as the

"Meningitis Belt," and outbreaks occur regularly during the dry season.[1] In the past, 80-plus percent of outbreaks were Meningococcal meningitis type A, but increasingly other serogroups have emerged: C, W135, Y, and even X. Although the treatment for all types of bacterial meningitis is the same, vaccine prevention is specific to the serotype. Widespread vaccination campaigns undertaken by the World Health Organization against type A have dramatically decreased reported cases and deaths in the past few years, but the other strains continue to spread.

My driver Nixon and I spent the next several weeks driving around Amudat District, population 180,000. I loved reciting the names of the villages: Nakapiripirit, Namalu, Nakaale, Tokora, Lorengedwat (Nixon's favorite), Nabilatuk and Moroto. I'm sure neither *The Rough Guide* or *Lonely Planet* lists them as highlights, or even mentions them at all.

Twenty years before I went to Amudat with MSF, my long-time roommate worked in the nearby sub-county of Namalu. A naïve young woman from small-town America, her job was to distribute school supplies from this remote Ugandan village. For years, I'd heard her stories about branches with three-inch thorns being used for fences, cattle with horns so big that holding their heads up must be nearly impossible, a headmaster being buried up to his neck in the schoolyard for some perceived slight, anthills taller than a person, and red clay soil that turned into a skating rink in the rain. I was thrilled to walk her same paths twenty years later, although Namalu was now a village struck by meningitis.

We left the relative comfort of the MSF compound and

moved into a Catholic mission inside a more centrally accessible village. Although the new compound was infested with mosquitoes, lacked running water, and served drab food, it had solar power, a generator, and was large and private. We took bucket showers at night, washed our clothes in the grey water, and brushed our teeth with boiled water in a recycled altar wine bottle. There was an "internet café" in our new hometown, but there was no internet. The best restaurant was a stick hut with dirt floors which served 50-cent breakfasts and one-dollar dinners. Beer was served warm because there was no fuel for the generator to run the cooler.

As an expatriate, it's always fun to explore markets for locally-produced items. My favorite item was a toilet paper brand appropriately named "Relax." The sights and sounds were so different from those at home: children in ragged dirty clothes screamed and cried to see my white skin and blue eyes but stopped crying upon seeing a balloon, behaviors like public nose-picking, which would be a social taboo at home, were common here, and babies were wrapped in bright fabric across their mothers' backs with their feet sticking out around their mother's waist. A two-year-old proudly tied her dolly onto her back with a towel.

Local medical facilities were rudimentary at best. The health units were tidy, yet there were serious sanitation issues without hand-washing stations or running water. Local nurses had closed-cropped hair typical of the local style and wore little white nursing caps that looked like muffin cups perched on their heads. I marveled at their always crisply pressed uniforms, knowing the process involved carrying water from a great distance, washing clothes by hand, hanging them to dry and finishing with hot charcoal inside a metal iron. Flies deposit their larvae on drying clothes and are only killed by high heat, otherwise the larvae burrow into the skin and cause severe infections. Jiggers and pigworms burrow into feet and need to be dug out before the larvae hatch.

Life expectancy here is thirty-seven.

Nixon drove me around to do case management, which meant making sure sick patients got proper treatment at the five designated treatment centers. In addition to managing medical needs, I was also an administrator and logistician. My budget was 3 million Ugandan shillings, which sounds like a lot until it is divided by 1800 to one US dollar (the exchange rate at the time), so it wasn't really all that much.

One of my most important tasks was to visit the small health units daily, gather information, and create a "line list" of patients. A line list details the history of an outbreak and pinpoints specific villages where a disease is most prevalent. I distributed meningitis treatments, oily chloramphenicol and ceftriaxone, along with printed treatment guidelines and injection supplies. It's a really interesting process to be at the start-up of an emergency project.

I faced challenges from the beginning. On day one, I got into an argument on the phone with the Minister of Health and the World Health Organization representative concerning dosing for oily chloramphenicol. After a couple of hours, they called back to change the dosing protocol and still had it wrong.

These health leaders need to know exactly what they are doing. When they don't step up, people die. They insisted they were correct and resented suggestions to the contrary. They were so adamant that the doctor from UNICEF stated the Ugandan Ministry of Health had achieved "over 100% coverage" in a previous vaccination campaign. You don't have to be medical to see the error.

In order to request the correct vaccine to stop this outbreak, spinal fluid needed to be collected from a dozen patients, analyzed, and the causative bacteria determined. Given the constraints of distance, and the lack of laboratory facilities and proper sample transportation, this crucial step can take up to two or three weeks. Once the predominant strain of meningococcal meningitis is identified, a request for vaccines is sent by the WHO to the international vaccination repository in Geneva.

While we at MSF provided daily case management to treatment facilities, we also began to design a vaccination campaign pending results of the causative agent. In an outbreak setting, meningitis vaccines are normally given to people from ages six months to thirty years if the previous vaccination coverage was inadequate. Among the Pokot tribe, vaccination coverage was zero.

Giving shots would be the easy part, but reaching people who needed the vaccinations would be a challenge. Vaccine distribution meant targeting about 130,000 people scattered across 1,600 square miles. Small pockets of people lived a six-hour climb up into the mountains with no road. We also worried that the outbreak would spread north and east to Kenya along with the wandering tribes.

MSF began to mobilize freezers, ice packs, vaccine carriers, and vehicles, always the heaviest part of a vaccination campaign.

This was a huge task, but no one stepped up to help us — not the District Health Office, not the Ugandan Ministry of Health, not the World Health Organization. MSF alone was leading the charge. And all the local actors looked to us for guidance. MSF has done this so many times in so many places that the organization has written guidebooks on how to deal with epidemics like meningitis and made videos about organizing and implementing mass vaccination campaigns.

Corruption became the biggest obstacle to the vaccination campaign strategy's success.[2,3] A daily "allowance" of $2 was budgeted over and above a person's regular salary. Without that "top up," no one would participate in the campaign. The district hospital's Cold Chain Manager (the person in charge of the freezers, refrigerators, and ice packs – essential for preserving integrity of vaccines) refused to cooperate during the vaccination campaign unless he received the additional "allowance" even though he would be doing his regular job and nothing more.

"It's a campaign," he said.

"Yes, but it's your regular job," I explained.

"But it's a campaign," he repeated.

The real reason for greed and corruption during vaccination campaigns is because money for interventions comes from large agencies like WHO and UNICEF. These agencies depend on UN funding but don't provide the actual hands-on care; they fund it. Everyone puts their hand out for their piece of the pie. But when MSF is involved, things are done openly, honestly and "by the book." MSF funding is independent of any other agency or government. There are no hidden agendas. There are no politics. There are no kickbacks. All populations are treated equally.

As we coached the District Health Officer on creating a budget, I noticed his line item for bribes. "The politicians will want to be paid to support the efforts among their people," he explained.

I was frustrated to see people die as a result of such ridiculous behavior. Day by day, the outbreak expanded while money was funneled to politicians and people doing their routine jobs, leaving less for hiring vaccinators, purchasing supplies, undergoing training, and garnering community support.

On February 2, the Ugandan groundhog must have stuck his head out of his burrow, seen corruption, and gone back inside forever.

Although the outbreak began in December, when WHO and UNICEF (provider of vaccines and funding) finally arrived that day amid much fanfare, the local authorities uninvited MSF to the party. They knew that if MSF was involved in strategy and implementation, they wouldn't be able to stretch out the response timeframe in order to ask for more money for "allowances." Population figures, especially in mobile societies like the Karamajong and Pokot, are always difficult to estimate. By inflating those numbers, more money would be allocated per person. MSF would also provide accurate coverage data, not "over 100%" as previously reported by the authorities.

MSF pointed out flaws in the logic used in the planning and suggested a better way, but the pride of local authorities doomed the program to fail the people it was intended to help. The Ministry of Health along with WHO and UNICEF had been widely criticized for the delay in initiating a mass vaccination campaign. Without adequate laboratory confirmation, they proceeded to request vaccines against meningococcal meningitis strain A, typically the most prevalent serotype. They conducted the vaccination campaign only for the Karamajong. MSF offered to vaccinate the excluded Pokot tribe, but was denied authorization.

The letdown was almost overwhelming. It was difficult to walk away after weeks of sleepless nights and pushing ourselves to the edge. Had we at MSF been allowed to do our jobs well, this massive outbreak would have been avoided and no one would have ever known.

But it was a big outbreak, and it was reported widely in the press. The final numbers would be touted as perfect while people continued to die.

MSF continued to obtain spinal fluid samples for testing according to guidelines. Three weeks later, those results revealed a different serotype that was not covered by the vaccine given in the campaign. The outbreak lingered with more cases, more adverse sequelae, and more deaths — an illness that would have been vaccine-preventable if the correct measures had been taken.

Reference list:

1. Hayward, Peter. "African Meningitis Belt: 2006." *The Lancet*, May 2006, www.thelancet.com/journals/laneur/article/PIIS1474-4422(06)70435-5/fulltext.

2. Africa, Business Insider Sub Saharan. "Uganda's Health Minister Went Undercover in a Hospital to Investigate

Corruption Allegations." *Business Insider*, Business Insider, 18 Sept. 2017, www.businessinsider.com/ugandas-health-minister-went-undercover-in-a-hospital-2017-9.

3. Lewis, Maureen. "Governance and Corruption in Public Health Care Systems." *Center for Global Development*, vol. 72, Jan. 2006, doi:http://www1.worldbank.org/publicsector/anticorrupt/Corruption%20WP_78.pdf.

Luck Runs Out
John Fiddler

After years of working in Central Africa, it had become apparent to me (and probably everyone else, too) that I worked better in remote settings.

So when I landed in Bangui's M'poko airport about six months ago, I was already anticipating my next flight out and away. I nervously pushed my way through chaotic crowds and past steely-eyed customs officials. My ultimate destination was an additional four-hour flight to the far southeast interior of the Central African Republic.

Humanitarian workers in the country's capital had to fight more than just fevers and malaria. The bureaucracy could be vicious. Daily we heard of anonymous acts of violence. Danger dwelled in the ruins of decrepit colonial edifices and lurked in the eyes of a malnourished military.

All over the country there had been convulsions of religious and ethnic strife, the sequelae of old injuries. The battles between Muslim and Christian, nomad and sedentary, man and microbe all remained unresolved. Danger also lived in the remote towns and small villages, but at least there I had a better chance of getting to know its name.

Our base was situated in a remote location in the heart of Zemio, near its market. This town was swollen by an influx of refugees fleeing from the surrounding countryside and from the Democratic Republic of Congo, visible across the M'bomou river. The town was comprised of settlements strung from east to west along a four-kilometer road parallel to the river. Driving along this road you would see a Muslim quarter, a Congolese refugee village, open-air markets, a United Nations (UN) compound, and an old religious mission school. Our headquarters and the twenty-bed hospital we supported were located at the eastern end of the town. We also ran a small outpatient clinic midway, near the UN base.

The population here was a collage of the Christian majority, a Muslim minority, and the ubiquitous Peuhl — semi-nomadic herders who also follow Islam. These herders had many names and were easily distinguished by their dress. Usually armed with *armes blanches* [knives or bows and arrows], they, along with their cattle, were considered outsiders and troublemakers.

From our base, I was able to walk through the market and up the steep hill to the hospital in about fifteen minutes. A stone's throw from the hospital was the *piste* [airport] at the top of the hill. Flying in and out of here was quite spectacular. After the airplane taxied, it came to a halt across the road from the local police station. Here the *gendarmes* [police force] positioned themselves outside the ramshackle building, looking tough and smoking. Sometimes they sat with their pet monkey, tied by a string to a chair. They were armed with guns and controlled the entrance and exit on the eastern road into the town.

I tried not to mix too much with these armed actors (or the monkey), but for security reasons I needed to regularly check in and explain what we were doing. Although we had many accurate sources of security information, we needed to maintain a friendly rapport with the gendarmes and army folk. This town of 25,000 souls, underserved and distant from the politics of Bangui, had only about eight soldiers from the Forces Armeés Centrafricaines (FACA) and five gendarmes to keep the peace.

The main reason for our presence here was the Lord's Resistance Army, or LRA, a legendary, violent group operating in the bush. Shadowy and unpredictable, they frequently tethered their captured prisoners, demanding they act as porters and slaves under threats of death. They were feared and reviled. Because of them, thousands of residents had fled from the countryside to shelter in this town, and we were here to deliver medical care to all. We heard of numerous acts of brutal violence, robberies, and fatal hold-ups on the dirt roads that radiated out from here. The LRA was not the only malevolent group around.

That particular morning, I awoke for my second day in charge of the project. Yesterday we had said goodbye to our experienced project coordinator. Her replacement was due in a week, and I was in charge in the interim. My primary responsibility was the safety of our staff and patients. I had slept uninterrupted the night before with my walkie-talkie radio by my side. No one had called me. It was Tuesday.

"*Mon Chef* [my boss], did you hear the gunshots last night?" The guards were eager to tell me about it.

I did not. I was suddenly alert. I remembered that it was me — I was the security "responsible".

"Why didn't anyone call me on the radio? What happened?"

"There were gunshots last night. A group of young militia returning to the town were shooting into the air in celebration. They captured a group of known bandits."

I was slightly relieved that the shots were celebratory.

"They are being held prisoner in the mayor's house, but there are angry crowds."

It was a warm, bright morning. I was in charge. I felt a chill breath of unease.

Something was going on a couple of kilometers away in the west of the town. Some of our national staff there had radios and were communicating with the base from their homes. The crowds, they said, were out for blood.

One of our staff told me the rumor: "They have captured three notorious bandits responsible for a recent killing and stealing from the villages. One man says he recognizes them. They are the bandits that killed his family, burned them, and cut out and ate their hearts in front of him."

Shit.

One of our nurses called on the radio and said he was not going to open our small clinic on his side of the town. The atmosphere was too charged. There were armed mobs.

"The prisoners are Peuhl Muslims, the Christians want revenge. The whole Muslim community is under suspicion, and all groups are now arming themselves for protection."

Outside the compound, all was quiet. Nothing appeared different. I asked the guards to call me if there was any news. I needed to go to the hospital. I was glad it was all happening on the other side of town.

"Keep me updated."

The morning walk through the town center past the swamp and up the steep hill was the same as ever - no crowds, no excitement. I was with the pharmacist and two reliable national-staff nurses. We reached the top of the hill and jumped over a ditch into the hospital grounds. Semi-wild pigs rooted amongst the fallen mango leaves. There were no walls or fences here.

I had grown to love this place and my work. I was eager to start the day, but I still had an uneasy feeling.

We saw the usual small group of patients, mostly sick children, gathered on a bench outside the ward. A *secouriste* [nurse's aide] was already taking the vital signs. We talked to the night nurse to review the overnight report. As I stood outside the room where we did wound dressings, an unfamiliar young man in civilian clothes came over and asked if we could speak privately. He seemed very serious.

"Sure," I said.

"I am the assistant to the commander of the gendarmerie. You know there are three Muslim prisoners that were captured last night?"

"Yes, I heard."

"They were being held at the mayor's house. The crowds wanted to kill them."

"Yes."

"The crowd attacked them. They tried to break into the house. We have taken them from the mayor's house. They are now being held for protection in a cell in the police station, but they have been badly wounded." He pointed over at the building.

"Yes."Oh no, not *here*.

"The Chief wants to know if you can come with your nurses to the police station to tend to them?"

Damn! Why were they asking me this? A dangerous reality settled over my morning. These prisoners were now only a few hundred meters away. I felt the fever of a real-life dilemma in my head.

We were trained to stay away from potentially violent situations, and we demanded a weapon-free humanitarian space. I didn't want my staff or myself in the middle of a dangerous situation, and it sounded like this town was simmering to a boil. But I also believed that I should help those in great medical need. Who is better deserving of medical attention than badly injured prisoners who are the potential victims of a lynch mob? Once you are badly injured, you are no longer a combatant. You are a patient.

But this is what we do.

I performed the moral equation in my head.

"We will come," I replied. "I will take two nurses and we will come, but we will stay a short time to assess the wounded and fix what we can and then we must leave."

My nurse colleagues did not object. In fact, they appeared to think it was the right thing to do. We gathered gauze and scissors, dressing kits, and some bottles of saline. We headed on foot from the hospital over to the police station.

I noticed something I had never seen before; there was a line of six or seven uniformed men standing in a row across the road looking down the hill into the town. Usually these guys hung out like actors on a set, but not now. This was different, this was serious, I could *feel* it. They were holding guns, maybe a grenade launcher, I didn't look too closely. One learns never to stare at armed men. I knew I just needed to tend to the prisoners and leave. I glanced to my right down the hill. There was no screaming mob. Everything was calm. There was no visible danger at this time. I thought, "Let's get this done quickly."

We walked through the decrepit police station's open door and into a dark empty room with a desk and an open rear window.

"Where are the prisoners?"

The policeman unlocked a wooden door in the corridor to my left. He led out two scared men. They stood shivering and wide-eyed, shell-shocked, and I realized immediately that they were not mortally wounded. I saw round eyes staring through a lace veil of dark blood. One of them was bleeding from a deep wound to his scalp from a blade. The other…had some blood from cuts, I didn't even know from where.

We got to work. I started to wash the blood off the shorter prisoner. He sat down while we washed and dabbed. My colleague assessed the other. We had to be quick. I was nervous. We were washing. Tearing tape. The prisoners were mute.

Suddenly I heard the sound of shouting voices, then… *WHOOSH,* a huge explosion. Then gunshots.

Fuck.

We all crouched down. "What is happening?"

The gendarme beside me told me the military was shooting at an armed mob. They were coming for the prisoners. My mind was racing. I was in the middle of an attack.

I couldn't believe it. I had always been lucky in my missions. A little danger had always been a familiar companion. I always told my friends and family the risks were minimal. On my previous missions, I usually left right before — or arrived just after — security incidents. But now I was here, and I was in the middle of something terrible. Explosions. Gunshots. Was this really happening? Was I going to die in a ramshackle police station in a small town in a corner of the Central African Republic? This was not the way it was supposed to be. I didn't even know if I was scared, but I knew I wished this wasn't happening.

I turned to my nurse colleagues, "We can't stay here."

I looked at the two prisoners. They stood there with frozen faces, underlying pallor, and eyes round like targets. Their forms were becoming transparent in the dark of the room. I understood in that instant that we all knew what was going to happen to them.

I pressed some final gauze onto the gash on one prisoner's head; it didn't look neat, which bothered me. I like to do neat dressings.

"I'm sorry, but we have to go," I whispered to them, and to myself.

The shooting suddenly ceased, but the shouting of many angry voices got louder. They were coming closer.

It was time.

"I'm sorry."

We ran out.

A Lesson in Hierarchy
Ana Cheung

I arrived in Panama to volunteer with a reputable non-profit organization on a medical mission as a nursing student. I was looking forward to working with local communities through the organization's many health clinics. This organization would travel by boat with supplies, medications, and medical volunteers to provide free healthcare to remote coastal villages, which lacked access to routine or emergency healthcare.

This was not the first time that I had been out of the country. A decade earlier, I had served in the Peace Corps as an agroforestry agent in West Africa. I was excited that the medical mission would combine my passion for nursing and international work.

On arrival, a local volunteer picked me up at the airport and informed me that the medical team had left yesterday for a mission and some R&R on a nearby island. They would be gone for a week.

The volunteer coordinator in the US had not mentioned this scheduling change. I was disappointed, as I could only stay for two weeks and was eager to begin mission work. This seemed to be a waste of resources, since the organization in the US had charged more than $500 per week per individual for housing. Had there been better communication between the volunteer coordinator and team leaders, I would have at least been able to meet the group since they had been close enough to pick me up to join them during their R&R. In retrospect, I am quite certain that had I been a healthcare provider, I would not have been left behind for the first medical mission.

When I arrived at the dormitories, I was surprised at their disheveled state. I was met with dirty clothes and linen strewn across the floor and heaped in assorted corners, empty and partially filled water jugs, and stained, unmade bunk beds covered with scrubs. The toilet, sink, and bathtub were caked in mold as well as a fine layer of dust. Unfortunately, the former and current volunteers had not done any cleaning.

Perhaps there were reasons for the mess. The doctor and founder of the organization lived off-site. He never visited the volunteer rooms. The landlord was in a wheelchair, so he was unable to monitor the state of his rooms, as they were upstairs. The organization did not have a cleaning staff (understandably), but there were no cleaning supplies on hand either. Seeing that I had to stay in the dormitories for the next two weeks, I cleaned the bathroom with my personal supply of toilet paper and my bare hands.

While the rest of the team was away, I spent the first week working at an affiliated geriatric facility. Although I was disappointed that I had missed the first medical mission, I enjoyed working with the geriatric patients. At least my first week wasn't a total loss.

When the team returned at the end of the week, I met the group, which included two registered nurses as team leaders, a nurse practitioner, and a few medical residents. As it happened, I was the only nursing student and the only person of color.

Soon, the nurse practitioner invited me to a breakfast with the group, but my tight student budget didn't allow for excessive expenses. Subsequently, the group would go out to meals, drinking, dancing, and socializing on their own. This also included socializing in their own dormitory rooms with doors closed.

We were a small group. In my experience, the smaller the group, the tighter the bond. You can imagine how surprised that I was to feel so alone with such a small team.

This was quite a contrast from my Peace Corps experience. In the Peace Corps, whenever there were new volunteers or volunteers visiting from their villages, everyone would make the effort to at least introduce themselves and get to know each other a little bit. Hierarchy was not an issue, because the missions were organized and we all worked on an equal playing field.

By the second week, a sonographer, along with a medical technology director, had joined our crew. The organization had made sure that the mission coincided with their arrival. A group welcome dinner was planned for them and the nurse practitioner demanded that I clean some of the dormitory rooms. It is normal to pitch in for cleaning during missions, but I had already cleaned my 6-bed dormitory room when the group was out on their R&R trip, and I felt like I had already done my share. It was only fair for the other volunteers to help out as well.

It was interesting to watch the other healthcare professionals make great efforts to get to know the new members and invite them out on multiple occasions. The mission had become increasingly isolating, and I was beginning to feel intentionally ostracized.

By this point, the nurse practitioner had already thrown out all my water jugs, some of my clothes, and the packaged snacks I had on the floor. I was not at the dormitories when this happened. When I let her know that my belongings were missing, she refused to apologize or compensate me for the loss, since she assumed the items belonged to departed volunteers.

She had also borrowed dishes and silverware from the room in which I was staying for the welcome dinner. I inquired if she was going to return them, and she abruptly retorted that they *had* been returned. After dinner, I found the soiled pile of silverware and dishes in my room for me to clean.

Either way, with the arrival of the medical team, I was finally going to be able to participate in the mission work that I came to do. As we prepared for the clinics, the nurse practitioner began to order me around while we were packaging supplies, etc. She never asked or thanked—just barked. I was shocked and upset by her imposing presence and condescending speech, of which I was the only target.

I reported the situation to the team leaders, who promised to speak with the nurse practitioner but never did. In the middle of the second week, about a dozen registered nurses and nurse practitioner students, accompanied by a nurse educator, joined our group. I learned after the fact that one of the nurse team leaders made a point to tell them to be nice to me since "*Ana is having a hard time [adapting]*." This may be the reason why the team leaders never addressed the nurse practitioner, as they saw me as the problem, not her.

We traveled in two boats to the clinic sites—one more ragged and one more modern. The nurse team leaders always directed the registered nurses and students to the older boat, whereas the providers, founder, and medical technology director always rode in the more modern boat. When setting up and breaking down mobile clinics, all volunteers were expected to participate. However, it was always the registered nurses and students who did most of the work. Again, the medical residents, nurse practitioner, and nurse educator were nowhere to be found.

I was concerned about other things as well. In the Peace Corps, being culturally sensitive was an important part of our work, but on this mission, those standards were disregarded. Our orientation packet clearly stated that volunteers should dress conservatively out of respect for cultural standards. The nurse practitioner and nurse educator wore short-shorts and donned easily visible g-strings. When they were questioned about their culturally inappropriate dress, they said it didn't matter.

In the Peace Corps, we had volunteers of all ages, expertise and backgrounds, but we treated each other as equals. We spoke to each other respectfully, as fellow professionals. This mission fell desperately short of any reasonable expectations. I contemplated leaving the mission entirely, something I never considered during my Peace Corps service. Even though I was in my 30's, this was my first taste of *nurses eating their young.*

I could only surmise that the reason why these issues were not being addressed was that we were "paying customers." This organization, like many others, relied heavily on repeat volunteers who spent their money and vacations on these trips. It was in the best interest of the organization to keep providers happy so that they would return for future missions, thus keeping the missions running and the organization afloat. Sadly, the money that the volunteers provide sometimes dictates how much of their bad behavior is tolerated on mission, even at the cost of losing other potential volunteers.

At the conclusion of my stay, I met with the founder of the organization to share my negative interactions regarding the nurse practitioner. He was supportive during the conversation, and I wondered: if I had approached him earlier, would things be different? Maybe if I had arrived one day earlier to Panama and had the chance to bond with everyone during the first mission and R&R, the group might have been more welcoming. Either way, we were all adults, and this should not have happened at all, yet bullying within the healthcare system occurs every day—vertically, laterally, and perennially, as an ongoing nursing issue for the last several decades.

In a perfect world, an organization would set up some ice-breaker activities so that all volunteers would be encouraged to interact with each other, instead of breaking into hierarchal cliques. Since that time, I have volunteered at various free clinics as a nursing student and registered nurse, where all volunteers are valued and hierarchy is not part of the culture. If you're considering a similar experience, here are some tips: research the organization thoroughly via blogs and website reviews, ask for recommendations through your network, especially alumni, confront bullies and report to management as needed, or travel with a friend.

We cannot change the culture, but we can make sure that the culture does not change us. The lesson of hierarchy was an unpleasant one, but I am grateful for the opportunity to have volunteered with the communities of Panama, that I had the privilege and honor to do so. It showed me the kind of provider that I never want to become and the kind of provider I aspire to be.

Leave Your Prejudice at the Door
Amanda Judd

Lately, I've been reflecting on what it means to be female in a world where females are the most vulnerable of the vulnerable. The powerlessness of women seems more incontrovertible the more humanitarian work that I do. Women suffer unspeakable things in this world. We are universes unto ourselves, but we remain marginalized and disempowered.

But if you are willing to listen, inspiration often occurs in the most unexpected of places. It is a rare gift to be able to sit in the home of your patient and talk to them about their day-to-day life, but I had that privilege on a recent mission in India.

After we left the Araveli clinic, our caravan of vehicles stopped on a narrow road on the side of a hill, a cornfield and a stepwell below and a small village above. We walked up the steep cobbled road into the village of Khamoda, surrounded by green forests lush from the recent monsoon. Khamoda is so small and remote that it doesn't exist on any map. You can't Google it. The closest that you can get is a search for the Kumbhalgarh Wildlife Sanctuary that surrounds Khamoda. Eight families call the village their home.

This is where Mamta Bai lives.

We found our way up to her one-room home through a narrow staircase. Her goats seemed eager to visit with her and tried to weave their way into our group and up the stairs. She laughed and chased them away. Mamta Bai mentioned that she also had two dogs until a few days before when a jaguar came and stole them away.

Leaving our shoes at the door, we entered her home through swinging doors that stop a foot short of the top of the doorjamb, allowing an illuminating shaft of light to seep in. The clean, well-organized single-room house functioned as a living room, bedroom, and kitchen. Mamta Bai ushered us in, inviting us to sit on rugs on the floor and lean on the walls that resembled adobe.

They were actually coated with smooth cow dung, a technique reported to repel mosquitos and to remain cool in the summer and warm in the winter. You might think that they would smell awful, but they don't. As we sat down to talk, Mamta Bai stoked the fire of her smokeless *chullah* (cook stove) and began to prepare *chapatti* (flatbread).

Mamta Bai and her husband are both illiterate. She was born into the most disenfranchised of the castes in India: The Tribals. Considered lower in the caste system than the Dalits (Untouchables), they are the least likely to have access to healthcare, education, and other services. Illiteracy is common to the point that even handling money is a challenge, much less having a bank account. Being illiterate and impoverished would, in most cases, leave her subject to being subservient. But, this is not the case for Mamta Bai. In Khamoda and communities like it, the elders are all men and ultimately make the final decisions, but Mamta Bai's story is unique. Her given name is Mamta. Bai is added to convey that she is a respected elder. By all accounts, she is an outlier and uniquely empowered. All of the women in her village look up to her.

She is in her fifties now, but early in her marriage, she lost three children and, as a result, became infertile. In her community, it's common for a man to leave an infertile woman due to her inability to bear children, but Mamta's husband was different. He stayed.

Mamta became a surrogate mother to all the children in her community. While the group of us sat and talked, a few of Khamoda's children hung out just outside the door. Mamta proudly showed us the corn and soya bean that she had grown and explained that she would prepare extra food for any hungry child in the village. The faint scent of the wood fire filled the air as Mamta Bai began to knead and roll the dough for chapatti.

She explained that she had many jobs to do. A sly smile appeared on her face when she mentioned that women are better multitaskers than men. With only one man in the room to defend himself, it was agreed that she was correct. Mamta's husband is a farmer and does masonry work when he has the opportunity, and Mamta collects eleven large pots of water daily from the stepwell below the village. She carries those pots on her head to her home for cooking, drinking, and washing. She keeps the home and cares for the animals. Twice a week, she treks into the forest to collect firewood. It takes her five hours to collect enough wood to warm her home, boil water, and cook meals. This is a brave act considering that that the wildlife reserve surrounding her village shelters many predators, including jaguars, jackals, wolves, and bears—all of which Mamta runs into frequently.

We went around the room and introduced ourselves, announced whether we were married and whether we had children. The unmarried women quickly became a focus for her matchmaking. She was confident that she knew someone for a single woman in the group. She was curious that I only had one daughter; in rural India, it is of the highest importance to have a son. A daughter may be seen as a burden. Female infanticide, while illegal, is not uncommon. I explained that I was very happy with my daughter. She said that people in her culture would continue to have children until they have a boy. She looked at me with sympathy for my single-child state and said, "It is God's will."

There was a part of me that felt that this was also her way of coping with the loss of her own children. In a culture that values being married and having children above all else, her suffering must have been immense.

Mamta Bai believes that education is the only way for children to change their station in life. She believes that she will always be illiterate, but she wants more for the children of Khamoda. If she finds out that a child is not in school, she will confront the family and shame them into putting the child back into school. Confrontations like this could be very dangerous for a woman, but Mamta Bai is not afraid. She knows that this is the only way to escape the grinding poverty and challenging life of the people in her village. Her influence is felt throughout Khamoda. When Mamta Bai does something, people follow.

In the US, we use a scale called an ACE (Adverse Childhood Experiences) score to determine an increased risk for depression, heart disease, cancers, alcoholism, violence, and additional factors detrimental to the health and quality of life for children.[1] ACE scores are ranked based on experiences of verbal abuse, physical abuse, neglect, and other similar circumstances. The higher the ACE Score, the more likely a child is to experience the negative effects of toxic stress.

But there is another scale of equal importance: The Resilience Score. The Resilience Score is based on numerous factors, including feelings of love and support and the existence of structure during childhood. Many of these experiences are reliant upon the external influence of one or more people. There is debate as to whether resilience is acquired through external forces or is based on one's inherent wiring, but either way, it can negate the impact of a high ACE score.

Certainly, Mamta Bai, as a Tribal and a childless woman, had all of the cards stacked against her. In my brief time with her, I never learned who influenced her resilience. Not only has she prevailed, she has become a leader in her own community and a person who will affect permanent generational change for the young girls and boys growing up there.

I began to rethink my own prejudice that stemmed from western culture, and I realized that it wasn't just my *shoes* that I needed to leave at the door. Empowerment looks different for everyone, but it is undeniable that Mamta Bai is a strong and powerful woman. Years later, as I walked through a crowd of women during a mission in Guatemala, I had to pause for a minute to remember that things are not always as they appear on the surface. I greeted all of the women patiently waiting to be seen. I thought to myself, "I bet there's at least one or two Mamta Bai's in this crowd."

Reference list:

1. "Got Your ACE Score?" *ACEs Too High*, 9 Apr. 2018, acestoohigh.com/got-your-ace-score/.

Education: A Catalyst for Change
Karly Glibert

*"Education is the most powerful weapon
which you can use to change the world."*
– Nelson Mandela

When I think about education and its profound impact, I think about my friend, Kennedy Daniel, who I met on my first trip to Malawi. I was twenty years old and trying to figure out what I had just gotten myself into by coming to the third world country of Malawi, Africa on a whim. Malawi is a place of poverty—typically ranked in the top ten, if not the top five, of the poorest countries in the world, depending on the source and year.[1] It is one thing to read a statistic and another to live in it. Despite this, I wanted to help in whatever way I could. In 2012, I was traveling with Circle of Hope International, which sends American teams to a place called The Grace Center in Malawi every summer. It was my first time in Malawi, but it would not be my last.

The Grace Center is a compound dedicated to community

development with a school, church, orphanage, textile center, clinic, and farmland. The drive from the airport to the center weaves through areas of open land littered with trees and mountainous backdrops and market areas bustling with people selling produce, clothing, or baskets. We pass by village after village composed of small mud or brick homes and roaming goats and chickens. At last, we arrive at a stone gate where there is a sea of adults and children ready to greet us. Returning team members are reunited with old friends in singing, laughter, tears, and hugs. Meanwhile, first-time travelers have no trouble finding barefoot children to hold their hands and guide them up the path to the official welcome party. Teams live at The Grace Center, sleeping on small foam mats in tents. We often wake up to the sound of a rooster's crow even if it is 3 a.m. and clearly not time to wake up yet. We have nicknamed our bathroom the "squatty potty" because it consists of a little hole in a concrete floor in a small wooden structure. For our daily bath, we get a bucket of water and use a smaller cup to pour the water over our heads. We use baby wipes to clean our dirt-stained feet before climbing into our sleeping bags at night, and if we get sick, we have an old white 15-passenger van that will whisk us off to the nearest clinic for treatment. Even in our simplicity, we live luxuriously compared to most Malawians.

That first summer, I was a student nurse and had prepared health lessons that I hoped would be helpful for a team of locals dedicated to learning basic first aid for those in the community. Each member of the Community Health Evangelist (CHE) team received a binder of lessons with pictures and translated words. The team was already helping ill community members with chores such as laundry and cooking, but they wanted to do more. The lessons were not as successful as we had hoped. We had underestimated the prevalence of illiteracy and how little Malawians knew about the most basic functions of the body; we had to be flexible. We quickly simplified, changed teaching tactics, and encouraged more interaction and visuals to make progress that summer.

Kennedy Daniel, the head of the CHE, sat at the back of each class and was always attentive. A decade my senior, he was usually quiet, but when he did speak, it was obvious that he had the respect of his peers. I don't recall Kennedy speaking a single word of English to me that summer. In fact, as we would walk to surrounding villages to share our health lessons with locals, we would do our best to communicate through pointing and gesturing. He would point to something just off the narrow dirt path created by the many feet that had passed before us and say the Chichewa word, waiting for me to repeat it. He never gave the impression that he understood what I was saying, and he always waited for the translator to interpret my words before responding. Yet, somehow, I walked away that summer feeling like I had a friend. We were partners, united in heart, with similar goals of improving the health of the community through clinics and preventative education. Kennedy, along with the people of the CHE, help to run the clinics, provide health education, offer first aid, and do home visits. When I returned for a second trip in 2013, you can imagine my surprise when Kennedy began casually speaking to me in semi-full English sentences — he had known English the whole time! We both still chuckle about that.

In 2013, I began to learn more about Kennedy. By that time, I had gained his trust, and he had gained mine. Kennedy's wife also works at The Grace Center in the summer, washing the clothes of American team members. She carries the clothes to the river to wash them before hauling the heavy, soaking loads back up the hill to our camp base to line-dry. At the time, they had two young daughters; the elder shares Kennedy's wide, round eyes and broad white smile. They now have an infant son, born in November of 2017. Kennedy and his family live in Katengeza village and, unlike most Malawians, Kennedy is not living in the village he was born into. He was informally adopted into Katengeza as an orphaned teenager when a man from the local church, Mr. Jonamu, agreed to take him into his home.

Before working at The Grace Center, Kennedy made cane chairs by the side of the road with Mr. Jonamu. To this day, Kennedy is considered Mr. Jonamu's son in Katengeza village, which is just a 5-minute walk from The Grace Center where he now leads the CHE. He is smart, has a desire to learn, and has the confidence to apply his new knowledge to his work. At times, Kennedy moves slowly because of pain from a broken ankle that was never treated properly. The injury left him with a visibly deformed joint that aches daily as he walks from village to village to provide care and education to the community. He serves in the praise band at church, both as a drummer and a singer.

Kennedy also has a good sense of humor. He likes practical jokes, such as saying "mwadzuka bwanji" (good morning/how did you sleep?) at 2 p.m. to see if I catch his mistake and respond with the correct Chichewa phrase for the afternoon. Once, he roared with laughter when I jumped up and squealed trying to get away from a cockroach.

Kennedy loves people and wants to alleviate the suffering he sees in his community, suffering that he has witnessed firsthand throughout his lifetime, suffering that has taken family and friends from him. One afternoon, sitting on the dusty concrete steps of the clinic, Kennedy shared his backstory and his testimony of God's faithfulness in his life with a small group of Americans and Malawians. As a part of his testimony, he shared that he had lost both his mother and his father as a teenager, one of whom he lost to cholera — a disease we had taught the CHE team about a few days prior.

Cholera is caused by bacteria that is usually passed through contaminated food and water. It is an important topic to cover due to its prevalence in Malawi. The disease causes extreme amounts of watery diarrhea that can rapidly dehydrate a person — quite literally — to death. The bacteria are carried in the fecal matter of those infected; therefore, good hygiene after using the toilet and before preparing food is essential.

In 2013, our lessons covered how to ensure safe food preparation and clean water source maintenance. We discussed prevention techniques, such as washing and storing dishes off of the ground, personal hygiene, and latrine systems that inhibit the runoff of stool into water sources. We taught people about the need for oral rehydration solutions, which provide necessary electrolytes, instead of rehydrating with water alone. I demonstrated by filling a bottle of water with a single cherry drink mix packet. The bright red color of the liquid represented the valuable electrolytes the body needs to survive. I poured the red liquid out of the bottle, little by little; it splattered off the hard dirt onto my feet. Each splatter represented the loss of fluid and electrolytes as a person has diarrhea. When the bottle was almost empty, I refilled it with just water, which is the way most Malawians would rehydrate. The bottle became full, but the liquid was extremely diluted and light pink. The visual example resonated with the CHE, and they took all that they learned about prevention and treatment to the surrounding villages while we were there and long after we had left.

Fast-forward three years to 2016, my third trip to The Grace Center. Kennedy and I were asked to do an interview for a video project reflecting on the progress we have seen over the years as a result of our education efforts. We sat down in front of a concrete wall in cane chairs — the same kind Kennedy used to make by the side of the road. We did not know what the interview questions would be ahead of time, and everything seemed ordinary, until it wasn't. As he responded to a question, Kennedy casually mentioned that he had not heard of a single case of cholera in the surrounding community since 2013 — the year we taught the CHE about cholera prevention. Suddenly, I forgot I was being filmed. My jaw dropped. Eyes wide, I quickly interjected, "WHAT?" He leaned forward in his chair and turned his head toward me; we locked eyes. He was speaking directly to me instead of to the camera now, repeating his words in Chichewa so as not to be misunderstood. The translator interpreted his statement the same way — he had not heard of cholera in the surrounding villages since 2013. I was overcome with a rush of thoughts and emotions. The information consumed my mind for the remainder of the interview.

He had not heard... of a single case of cholera...
in the area... since 2013.

I felt a range of emotions: disbelief, joy, excitement, and even sorrow. Sorrow? Yes, sorrow. When I recounted the story to teammates later that day, my eyes welled with tears and my lip quivered. I couldn't shake the question: "It is so simple, why didn't anyone tell them sooner?" I will never get a satisfactory answer, so I choose to rejoice in the fact that they *do* know now. The immediate and obvious difference in the community is almost unbelievable. The results are beyond what we as a team ever anticipated. We can see that our partnership is making a difference; education is making a difference. The observable change in the community has only reinforced the community's trust in the information we bring them, so we continue educating.

We continue to hold our pop-up clinics, where we treat acute illnesses during the summer months when Americans are present. However, these clinics are just "putting out fires" and we would rather prevent the fires. Because of this, we have been intentionally incorporating health education into our programs in as many ways as we can. We have continued health education for our CHE and held special classes for mothers, teens, and children. Through our lessons and programs, we have seen improvement in the severity of infected wounds, a reduction in malnutrition in the community, and more. Education, passed on from one person to another, reaches more villages and more people than we could reach individually during our short trips, leaving the longest-lasting impact.

We have a long way to go and many dreams about what the health of the community will look like in the future. We dream of a clinic that will run full time on The Grace Center campus. We dream of classes that are taught year-round for expectant mothers and mothers of small children. We dream of growing our current school by one grade each year until we have a university — a university that will educate the next generation of Malawians.

When I started this journey, I had the mindset of "What can I do to help?" With time and experience, my question has shifted to "What can I do to enable you to help yourself?" Most of the time, I have found the answer to this question to be to involve community health care workers like Kennedy with the education process in order to ensure that education continues when we are not there. Now, as I look both backward and forward at the same time, I realize that education is the indispensable tool required to accomplish all we hope and dream for Malawi.

Reference list:

1. *Malawi.* International Monetary Fund, July 2017, www.imf.org/~/media/Files/Publications/CR/2017/cr17184.as hx

Writing

Lang Leav

There is one thing you should know about writing. It
will inevitably lead you to dark places as you cannot write
authentically about something unless you have lived it.
However, you should always bear in mind that you are only
a tourist and must remain one. You were blessed with
the gift of words, in order to bring a voice to suffering. But
do not be too indulgent despite how addictive sadness can be,
how easy it is to get lost down the path of self-destruction. You
must emerge from adversity, scathed but victorious to tell your
story and, in turn, light the way for others.

Luz Maria
Monserrat Dieguez

"Education breeds confidence. Confidence breeds hope.
Hope breeds peace." - Confucius

Luz Maria comes from a village called Sajquiyes, northwest of
Guatemala City in the department of San Juan Sacatepequez.
Even though she grew up in a rural area of Guatemala, she was
lucky enough to receive an education in Guatemala City. I say
"lucky enough" because in Guatemala, simply being Mayan
attracts racial discrimination despite the twenty-two different
ethnicities present in the country.

Being Mayan and a girl can mean an entire life doomed to hard
work, no sense of self, and becoming a baby-making machine at a
very young age. Despite the odds, with the help of her great aunt,
Doña Teresa, Luz was lucky enough to receive an education. Doña
Teresa was able to escape from the civil war that occurred in
Guatemala from 1960 until the peace agreement in 1996. The war
lasted 36 years and was the longest civil war in Central America.
Over 200,000 Indigenous people were massacred in the genocide.

Many more people simply disappeared.

During the war, Doña Teresa was resourceful, and she was able to find a job as a maid in a rich family home. Eventually, after years of hard work, she found a job selling flowers at "The Terminal", a stall in the main market of Guatemala City. The job was a perfect fit for Doña Teresa; she came from San Juan Sacatepequez, known as the city of flowers due to the many varieties of flowers found there.

Doña Teresa was always amazed that Luz Maria could speak, read, and write both Spanish and Kaqchiquel, the Mayan language that is spoken in the area of San Juan Sacatepequez. At almost seventy years old, Doña Teresa still had difficulties writing her own name.

Luz Maria always showed great determination and begged her mother to let her finish elementary school. School was a challenge, especially considering that Luz had six siblings and, on most days, ate only one plate of rice and beans. School is difficult when you're hungry and even more difficult when no one is able to help you with homework. Luz's parents did not speak Spanish—the official language—and were illiterate.

Doña Teresa knew something had to be done so that Luz Maria could continue her education and maybe even obtain a college degree. Doña Teresa had seen on television that Indigenous women were becoming doctors and lawyers— something that she never could have imagined possible and would not have believed without seeing for herself. So, Doña Teresa gathered her courage and explained her plan to Luz's parents: She would bring Luz to Guatemala City to finish school, and in turn, Luz would help her in the market after school. Doña

Teresa explained that she was tired and truly needed to pass on the market job to a relative, but only to a relative that was smart enough. Doña Teresa had to do this while teaching Luz the business of flower sales; it only made sense to have Luz Maria come to Guatemala City! Luz's parents were hesitant, but after a while, it didn't seem like such a bad idea. After all, it was no additional expense for them; Doña Teresa would be taking care of everything. "One less mouth to feed," thought Luz's dad.

As the years went by, Luz lived in the city. She became aware of the challenges in her country, as well as their impact on her because of her ethnicity and gender. Luz became the first person in her entire family to graduate from high school. She came to realize that there was no profession for her other than teaching. Afterwards, in spite of Doña Teresa efforts to convince Luz to stay in the city and find a well-paying job, Luz decided to go back to her village and become a preschool teacher.

When Luz arrived home, she found out that a principal in Montufar village had renovated the old school and was developing a Spanish program for preschoolers so that upon arrival into elementary school, the students wouldn't encounter a language barrier. If the children were fluent in Spanish, their chances of dropping out of school would lessen. Fewer children would be in the fields, and the cycle of poverty could eventually be broken.

Both valuing the importance of teaching kids the Spanish language while still retaining their indigenous roots, Luz and Professor Rene—my Dad—got along perfectly. But life being life, after three years of hard work, young Luz got a hernia in her stomach. She was only twenty-three years old. A stomach hernia is operable, but Guatemala is a post-war country and corruption has made health care into a deplorable situation. After being placed on a waiting list in the Guatemala City Public Hospital with an estimated wait time of six to eight months, Luz thought about turning to a private hospital. But she would need about Q12,000 (around $1,700), which was totally out of the question.

The hernia was growing. The discomfort made teaching impossible, and since there was no substitute teacher, the preschool had to be shut down until further notice. There were many things in life that Luz felt she could face, but letting her students down was not going to be one of them.

One day, Luz was coming back from Guatemala City, where she had been rejected for a loan to pay for the hernia surgery. She was feeling down when someone on the bus handed her a flyer. It said something about a *jornada* with affordable medical, dental, and surgical care in San Raymundo, which was about thirty minutes from her village. Luz heard someone speaking on the back of the bus, saying that the surgeries were affordable, but one needed to arrive very early to receive a number and eventually be seen and evaluated by the medical team.

Luz was determined. She approached the lady on the bus and asked *how* early. The lady responded that Luz would need to be there as early as a day before.

Luz had saved Q1500, and she asked her Great Aunt, Doña Teresa, for another Q500. She had a total of Q2,000 (about $280). A week later, she got together with the people from her village. They rented a pickup truck so that they could get to San Raymundo hospital where the *jornada* would begin the following day. When they arrived on Saturday at eleven pm, there were already about ten people making a line. Numbers were not going to be given out until Sunday around five am.

Luz is a light and a beautiful spirit. From the Q500 she had borrowed from Doña Teresa, she bought meat, beans, rice, and tortillas, and she made a *carne asada* (or barbecue) for everyone outside while they waited.

She eventually got her number.

I met her while translating for the nurse practitioner who was evaluating her before she saw the surgical consultant. While we were talking about the food she had made for everyone waiting patiently overnight in the cool mountain air, she said to me, "We needed to stay warm, but making a fire without *carne asada* did not make sense!" I could see her eyes light up with excitement.

For Luz, the surgery was a celebration. It meant that she was going to be able to start where she had left off with her students. It meant that generations of bilingual first graders would be able to understand their textbooks and help translate for their parents—and maybe even teach them the language!

After Luz Maria fully recovered, I heard from my dad, Professor Rene, that even though the school year was over, she had asked for a classroom to finish teaching the preschoolers. Once my dad agreed, Luz went to the students' houses one-by-one to speak to their parents. She explained that she was healthy and ready to finish teaching the children so that they could move to first grade the following year.

Luz Maria. The exact translation for the name is "Maria's light." Luz's light was almost turned off by her life circumstances, but because of others, that light was not extinguished. When people decide to bring their own light into other people's lives, it is bright enough to make the hopeless darkness go away.

Reader's Guide

- Humanitarians sometimes begin their work later in life, as in Liza Leukhardt's "African Skies." Do you feel that there should be an age limit for humanitarian workers, or do you feel that life experience would enhance patient care in these situations? Defend your position.

- "The Road of Good Intentions" describes culture shock, religious proselytization, and orphanage tourism. What can you do prior to traveling to help prevent culture shock? Do you think it is appropriate for medical organizations to try to convert their patients? Do you think that it is appropriate to go to other countries to work with orphans after learning that many times "orphans" have parents and that this is many times a money-making scheme? In what ways does this type of work put orphans at risk? What would be a better way to support these children? Defend your position.

- In "The Problem with Little White Girls (and Boys): Why I Stopped Being a Voluntourist," Pippa Biddle describes being an unskilled volunteer going into countries where she was expected to build a library and care for HIV+ children. What impact do you think volunteering without appropriate training or education has on the efficacy of a mission? How do you think having ethnic, cultural, or language barriers impacts your objective? Defend your position.

- It is time-consuming to establish an effective long-term mission. In "The Burden" by Dianne Thompson, the mission developed over years. Would you consider committing to long-term mission work? Do you think that long-term mission work is more effective than short-term? Why or why not? Can these different types of work complement each other? When the 8-year-old girl died from her burden of worms, it was likely due to a diagnosis that came too late. What responsibility do you have as a humanitarian worker to educate yourself on the conditions you may encounter in the region you are working? What will you do to learn about conditions you may not encounter at home before you leave?

- In "The Story of a Birth: Zambia, Africa," Devorah Goldberg explores the challenges of working in a resource-poor environment. What adjustments do you think are necessary to provide care in a resource-poor environment? How much are you willing to adjust your standard of care to maintain quality care in this type of environment? Are you willing to competently work outside of your comfort zone?

- In "Approach and Landing," Elise Peterson explains that with a properly planned mission you can gain confidence and inspiration as a nurse. How has humanitarian work changed you? Has it made you a stronger provider? Defend your position.

- Sometimes poorly planned missions result in poor standards of care. "Do No Harm" discusses issues of medical competency and the questionable ethics of organizations. What questions will you ask before you go on your next mission? Why? Will you request a formulary? Would you want to know where you are staying? Do you want to know your team mates' qualifications and training? What will you do if you do not get adequate answers from the organization with which you are planning to travel?

- In "Trust Your Gut," Emily Scott discusses working in an Ebola zone with a well-respected organization. What risks are you willing to take to care for patients in an area with a high risk of infection? How much protection against illness is your responsibility? How much responsibility does the organization with which you travel bear? What are your options if your organization does not provide a safe working environment?

- In many parts of the world, there is increasing awareness of the impact of sexual assault and abuse, yet there is little in the way of legal recourse or social services to assist the victims of these crimes. In "The Suffering Grass," Amanda Judd discusses a young girl who was being assaulted. How would you have handled the situation differently? Do you think it is appropriate to step in to alter the course of a situation in a culture that is not your own? If you took action, do you think it would have a positive or negative impact on the victim?

- In "Follow the Money," Sue Averill explores the complex world of humanitarian aid and the funding of such ventures. What barriers do you expect to encounter while doing humanitarian work? How will you respond if you are unable to provide care and lives are lost due to these barriers? Averill describes the Ugandan Ministry of health stating that they achieved "over 100% coverage" in a recent measles vaccination program. Do you think that it is appropriate to be a whistleblower in cases of unethical work? What impact do you think that will have?

- In "Luck Runs Out," John Fiddler has the difficult and sometimes dangerous task of providing humanitarian care in a conflict zone. Do you think that neutrality is an important cornerstone in humanitarian work? Do you think that the nurses should have cared for the patient, possibly risking their own lives? What do you think the outcome would have been had they stayed with the patients? What would you have done had you been in charge of that situation? Defend your position.

- Sometimes, situations are different than they may appear when looking through the lens of western eyes. "Leave Your Prejudice at the Door" describes one of these situations. What prejudice or prejudgments do you think that you carry when traveling outside of your culture? Do you think that being an empowered person is a characteristic exclusive to western cultures?

- Many times on mission, you will find a skilled and experienced surgeon mopping floors. As a humanitarian worker, should you be willing to help out with jobs such as cleaning and sterilization that are not part of your job at home? Why? In "A Lesson in Hierarchy," Ana Cheung describes volunteers who are inappropriately dressed. Do you think that team leaders have a responsibility to step in when members of the team are dressing or behaving in a way that is culturally inappropriate?

- Cholera is a disease that is preventable with precautionary measures and education. In "Education: A Catalyst for Change," Karly Glibert discusses how cholera education prevented outbreaks of this disease in a community. What other diseases might be prevented by education? How will you implement this education on your next mission?

- In "Luz Maria," Monserrat Dieguez tells the story of Luz, a remarkable patient who, as a result of mission work, was able to return to her village to continue teaching language to students and helping to negate the impacts of generational poverty and oppression. What impact would you like to have as a health care provider doing humanitarian work? What are you willing to do in order to make this possible?

Glossary

armes blanches: (French) thrusting weapon; bows and arrows.

bucket bath: a water-sparing method of bathing in water-scarce regions using 1-2 buckets of water.

build capacity *or* **capacity building**: process of strengthening infrastructures, skills, and resources over time.

carne asada: (Spanish origin) roasted or grilled marinated meat.

ceftriaxone: third-generation cephalosporin antibiotic with broad-spectrum coverage.

Chichewa: language spoken in the central and southern regions of Malawi as well as parts of Mozambique, Zambia, and Zimbabwe; part of the Bantu family of languages.

cholera: intestinal illness caused by the bacterium *Vibrio cholera* transmitted via the oral-fecal route causing severe diarrhea that kills 50% of affected people if untreated; also called "the blue death" due to the bluish hue the skin takes on with dehydration.

cold chain manager: individual in charge of insuring uninterrupted refrigeration or temperature control of vaccines or medication in a hospital or healthcare system.

formulary: list of available medications.

gendarmes: (French) armed police force.

grey water: wastewater without fecal contamination.

hazmat: hazardous materials.

hijab: (Arabic origin) veil or head covering worn by some Muslim women; often covers the head and neck to the tops of shoulders.

HIV: human immunodeficiency virus is a retrovirus that eventually develops into acquired immunodeficiency syndrome (AIDS).

huipil: (Nahuatl origin) traditional cotton garment worn by women of central Mexico to Central America as a blouse; frequently hand-woven and embroidered.

infant warmer: beds used in a nursery to maintain a neonate's body temperature and minimize the expenditure of metabolic body energy.

jiggers: parasitic insect found in the tropics; also called tunga penetrans, sand flea, chigoe flea.

jornada: (Spanish origin) term used in Latin America for a short-term medical mission that is often set up in temporary medical facilities that may include surgical, medical, or dental care at an affordable rate.

kala azar: (Assamese origin) a parasitic infection spread by infected sandflies causing weight loss, splenic and hepatic enlargement, fever, and anemia with a high fatality rate if untreated; also called black fever, visceral leishmaniasis, Dumdum fever.

Kaqchiquel: indigenous Mesoamerican language spoken by Mayans of the western highlands of Guatemala.

Karamajong: sub-Saharan pastoral herders from the Karamoja region of Uganda.

K'iche': indigenous Mesoamerican language spoken by Mayans of the western highlands of Guatemala.

kitenge: (Kiswahili origin) cotton fabric, typically with colorful designs of East African origin.

line list: epidemiological record keeping method that tracks the history of a disease outbreak and prevalence of disease in particular areas.

Maya/Mayan: indigenous ethnic group that traditionally occupies Mexico, northern Belize, Guatemala, and northern Honduras.

membranes: term used in reference to labor and childbirth meaning amniotic sac.

meningitis: inflammation of the meninges; causes may be viral, bacterial, fungal, or protozoan, with bacterial having the highest mortality rate.

mon chef: (French) my boss.

Médecins Sans Frontières (MSF): independent, international NGO that provides humanitarian and medical aid in conflict zones, neglected areas, natural disasters, and emergency situations; also called Doctors Without Borders in the US.

mwadzuka bwanji: (Chichewa origin) phrase meaning "good morning"/"did you sleep well."

oily chloramphenicol: cost-effective broad-spectrum antibiotic; may be used to treat meningitis, ocular infections, and more; may cause bone marrow suppression; also called chloramphenicol oil suspension.

piste: (French) path, in this context used as a runway for the airport.

Pokot: East African tribal group living in Kenya and Uganda.

Pott's Disease: a form of extrapulmonary tuberculosis affecting the vertebral joints, eventually causing vertebral collapse with neurological sequelae including paraplegia; also called Pott Disease, tuberculous spondylitis, spinal tuberculosis.

Red Zone: area in which the risk of contamination with infectious substances is the highest; also referred to as the hot zone.

responsable: (French) responsible.

secouriste: (French) rescue worker.

sequela(e): secondary effect of an injury, illness, or condition.

serogroup: bacteria or viral illness with a common or closely related antigen.

skin-to-skin: a method of regulating a neonate's heartbeat, breathing, and temperature without complex equipment; also called kangaroo care.

sonographer: a person who performs diagnostic ultrasounds.

suction: when used in reference to childbirth, aggressively and quickly establishing a vacuum in a baby's mouth, typically with a syringe bulb, in order to remove any amniotic fluid, meconium, or other foreign substances to ensure that the baby's airway is clear to breathe.

triage system: medical system used to determine the severity and urgency of an illness or injury; determines order of treatment.

tuberculosis: a highly-contagious bacterial infection that primarily affects the lungs; high mortality if untreated.

United Nations (UN): an intergovernmental peace and securities organization.

underserved: vulnerable populations that suffer from disparities in access to services such as healthcare.

UNICEF: a UN-sponsored program that provides humanitarian aid to children and mothers in developing countries; also called the United Nations Children's Fund.

World Health Organization (WHO): a United Nations sponsored program that has a primary function focusing in global health and international public health responses.

Acknowledgements

This book would not have been possible without the tireless work of humanitarian workers around the world and the fearless individuals willing to share their truths in these stories.

I would like to thank Sue Averill and One Nurse At A Time for your tireless commitment to giving back to the humanitarian community and putting more "nurse" into the world. This book would not exist without you.

I'd like to thank Lang Leav for lending us "Writing" — it gave me a guiding light on this journey. And, to Pippa Biddle, for your astute insight into voluntourism. Thanks to Sigma Theta Tau International for allowing ONAAT to reprint "The Suffering Grass."

I would like to thank William Judd for not being worried when I had decided to take off on a journey to places unknown — you were right, I went on that first mission and completely "fell in." Thanks to Aria because your existence has made me a better person every day. Much gratitude to Ashley Scott for having listened to me endlessly talk about this book.

I'd like to thank Hendrix College and all of the students in the Odyssey Program. Bailey Brya, Oliver Kuhns, Zelda Engeler-Young, Sarah Weems, Peyton Penny, Michelle DeLouise-Ashmore, Lily Bay, Jasmine Zandi, Leah Crenshaw, Jacie Andrews, and Peyton Coffman, your work has been invaluable. Dr. Tyrone Jaeger, many thanks to you for your generosity in organizing the Odyssey Program.

About the Hendrix College Odyssey Program

The Editorial Assistants for *Lessons Learned* are students at Hendrix College, and, under the supervision of Dr. Tyrone Jaeger, Associate Professor of English-Creative Writing, they completed their editorial tasks as part of an Odyssey Special Project.

A private liberal arts college in Conway, Arkansas, Hendrix College consistently earns recognition as one of the country's leading liberal arts institutions, and is featured in *Colleges That Change Lives: 40 Schools That Will Change the Way You Think About Colleges*. Its academic quality and rigor, innovation, and value have established Hendrix as a fixture in numerous college guides, lists, and rankings. To learn more, visit www.hendrix.edu.

In the fall of 2005, Hendrix College launched a bold new curricular initiative titled *Your Hendrix Odyssey: Engaging in*

Active Learning. The Odyssey Program coordinates all experiential learning under this curriculum. In order to graduate, all students are required to complete three Odyssey experiences, each from a different category: Artistic Creativity, Global Awareness, Professional and Leadership Service to the World, Undergraduate research, and Special Projects. Students may earn Odyssey credit through pre-approved courses, pre-approved activities or self-designed projects. Each experience has a faculty or staff sponsor on campus who works with the student.

Biographies

Sue Averill, RN, Co-Founder and President of One Nurse At A Time. Growing up as an Army brat gave Sue a love for travel and other cultures, which was cemented when she lived in Mexico for two years as a young woman. Sue wanted to be a nurse since she was five-years-old and started her ER nursing career in 1979. After a devastating earthquake in Mexico City in 1985, she organized and led a 21-person team that provided medical care to an affected area in collaboration with The Salvation Army — Sue's first foray into the humanitarian arena.

After obtaining her MBA and doing a stint in the business world, Sue decided to dedicate more of her time to humanitarian medical work: teaching in Cambodia, making surgical and medical trips to Asia, Africa, and Latin America, and helping to design medical clinics in Honduras and Vietnam. She now considers herself a "Humanitarian Snowbird" — enjoying spring and summer in Seattle and working for Doctors Without Borders and other volunteer organizations during the winter.

The key for Sue came during a surgical trip to Pakistan; in comparison to girls and women there, she has lived a charmed life. Sue was born in a time and place that fosters independence, education, and freedom for women. She believes it to be her responsibility to give of herself for the many gifts that she has received through no merit of my own. One Nurse At A Time grew out of frequent inquiries by others: "How can I get involved and do what you do?" ONAAT's goal is to make it easier for nurses to use their skills to help people around the world, to lower the entry barriers, and to increase public awareness of the role and contribution nurses make in the humanitarian world. Sue truly believes that we CAN change the world.

Pippa Biddle is a New York-based writer. Her work has been published by *Guernica, The Atlantic, Wired, BBC Travel,* and more. Her work on volunteer and service-based tourism has been featured in *The New York Times, The Independent,* and *Al Jazeera* and she is featured in the 2015 documentary *Volunteers Unleashed.* Pippa has appeared as a guest speaker at numerous universities, institutions, and events around the world and previously served as the Roots & Shoots Youth Leadership Fellow at the Jane Goodall Institute.

Ana Cheung is a registered nurse with experience in medical-surgical, home health, and fertility nursing. Prior to her career as a nurse, she served in the Peace Corps and worked in the nonprofit sector. She is currently pursuing her master's degree as a Family Nurse Practitioner and plans to work in a medically underserved community. In her spare time, she volunteers at free clinics. She is originally from Brooklyn but currently resides in Pennsylvania with her husband and cat.

Monserrat Dieguez was born in 1986 and raised in Guatemala City. Since the age of eight, she has studied English as a second language. She acquired a degree in Literature from Guatemala City University in 2007. From 2010 till 2013, Monserrat worked as a middle and high school teacher for the language arts. Her bilingual fluency enabled her to begin a career as an interpreter, and she has been interpreting for the past four years. Monserrat has a strong love for education and dedicates her spare time to working towards anything that can enhance people's lives for the better. Currently, Monserrat volunteers with the Biblioteca Lic. Bernardo Lemus Mendoza school, which seeks to break the cycle of poverty through education in Guatemala. (www.yo-o.org) Hopefully, Monserrat's dreams of being a nurse will soon come true. Monserrat lives in Guatemala City with her daughter, mom, and brother.

John Fiddler is a Nurse Practitioner born in Dublin, Ireland. He currently works as a Hospice and Palliative Care Consultant in New York City. He obtained his diploma in tropical medicine from the Royal College of Surgeons, Dublin Ireland, and has worked intermittently for Doctors Without Borders since 2005. He passionately believes in nursing, teaching, learning, writing, art, and activism.

Karly Glibert was born in Archbold, Ohio and obtained her BSN from Indiana Wesleyan University in 2014. She is an ICU nurse in Chicago, Illinois, where she resides with her husband. Karly serves on the board of directors for Circle of Hope International (www.cohcommunity.org) and is planning her fifth medical mission trip to Malawi, Africa, where she focuses on community health education and wellness checkups for local children. She is currently obtaining her master's in nursing education from Grand Canyon University because of her love for teaching and her strong belief that education is a catalyst for change.

Devorah Goldberg, BS, RN, is an Emergency Room nurse in New York City. Ms. Goldberg is a graduate student in the Adult Nurse Practitioner program at Hunter-Bellevue College of Nursing and received her baccalaureate degree in nursing from Adelphi University in 2013. When she is not in school or has time off work, Devorah enjoys combining her two passions: travel and nursing. Devorah enjoys traveling to countries that are rich in culture but lack certain basic medical availabilities so that she can contribute to medical interventions and gain a cultural learning experience as well. Devorah has blogged about some of her nursing adventures, including her travels, since she began her career in 2013. Instagram: @strivingnovice Blog:StrivingNovice.com

Amanda Judd, MSN-FNP, BSN, BA, Board Member One Nurse at a Time. Amanda is a Colorado-based nurse practitioner. She obtained her BA in Anthropology/Sociology from Rollins College and later received her BSN and MSN-FNP from the

University of Colorado at Colorado Springs. She began her nursing career as an ICU nurse, has worked in the ER, and currently works as a community/rural health provider. Since becoming a nurse, she has spent much of her career learning about global health and volunteering both at home and abroad. In her spare time, she loves traveling, exploring museums, hiking, and enjoying the beauty that surrounds us all.

Liza Leukhardt RN, BA, MS, recently retired from a gratifying twenty-five-year career as a hospice nurse. Having gone down many other career paths earlier in life, nursing led her to fulfill much of her bucket list, including volunteering for nursing missions in Africa, India, and South America. Although retired, nursing continues to be a vital part of her identity, and volunteering for nursing missions remains a passion. Currently she is lucky enough to live in a vibrant, noisy and thriving *barrio* in the northern Andes of Ecuador. She hopes to continue her volunteer work in Ecuador as long as her teammates are able to haul her onto the bus!

Elise Peterson MSN, MPH, BSN, CPN, is California-born but has lived in Michigan, Chicago, and Florida and now calls Denver home. On her good days she can be found attending outdoor concerts, road tripping, hiking trails, and scoping out the latest restaurants and food trucks. On her bad days she is busy getting to all 50 states in the US, plotting her next international adventure, and trying to make the world a better place for her niece and nephew. She is a proud Wolverine, Gator, and Ranger alumna. The best things in her career have been teaching nursing students, starting a legal career, being an international medical mission trip junkie, and thriving as a nurse in the Pediatric ICU and PACU with the kiddos.

Emily Scott is a Registered Nurse who has treated Ebola patients in Sierra Leone, worked with search-and-rescue teams in Nepal, and delivered babies in Haiti. She specializes in Labor and Delivery when she's at home and travels for humanitarian medical missions and disaster response as often as she can. Emily lives in Seattle, Washington with her husband and their rescue dog. She blogs about ethical travel and volunteering at www.twodustytravelers.com.

Dianne Thompson has been a registered nurse since she graduated from Asheville-Buncombe Technical College in 1988. She is a co-founder of the Boca Costa Medical Mission, now Partners in Development (www.pidonline.org), in Guatemala and has been a volunteer nurse for this mission since February, 2003. As a nurse, Dianne sees clients in hospital, clinic, and home settings. She coordinates their needs with services offered through the Boca Costa Medical Mission and refers clients to other services in the area. Dianne also teaches nursing skills to local health promoters.

Christine VanHorn, One Nurse At A Time Support Staff. When she was a child, her family thought it was important for them to travel as much as possible. Christine was able to see much of the U.S. and Europe but saw little of the needs of the rest of the world. As an adult, Christine has come to realize how lucky that she has been and how much she needs to give back to her community and to the world.

In addition to working full time as a Performance Improvement Coordinator, she has the privilege of serving in an administrative capacity for One Nurse At A Time. Christine cannot express how much that she enjoys reading about the work being done around the world by volunteers. She loves helping nurses reach their dreams of going on missions to help those in need of medical care who would not receive it otherwise. Every organization that she reads about in ONAAT's directory and every scholarship nurse report that she reads made her want to go on a mission trip as well.

Christine was fortunate to go on her first medical mission to Belize in 2014. She had the opportunity to see first-hand the needs of the world and the difference that nurse volunteers could make.